try it!

AUTOIMMUNE COOKBOOK

by Amari Thomsen, MS, RD, LDN

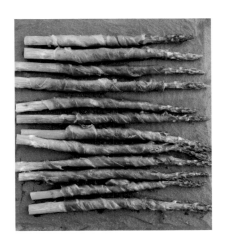

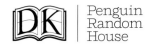

DK INDIA
Project Editor Arani Sinha
Art Editor Jomin Johny
Deputy Managing Editor Bushra Ahmed
Managing Art Editor Navidita Thapa
Pre-Production Manager Sunil Sharma
Senior DTP Designer Pushpak Tyagi
DTP Designers Nityanand Kumar and
Vijay Kandwal

DK UK
Angliciser Jamie Ambrose
Project Editor Kathryn Meeker
Senior Art Editor Anne Fisher
Design Assistant Rehan Abdul
Managing Editor Stephanie Farrow
Managing Art Editor Christine Keilty
Jacket Designer Amy Keast
Producer, Pre-Production Andy Hilliard
Producer Stephanie McConnell

First published in Great Britain in 2016 by
Dorling Kindersley Limited,
80 Strand, London WC2R 0RL

Copyright © 2016 Dorling Kindersley Limited
A Penguin Random House Company
15 16 17 18 19 10 9 8 7 6 5 4 3 2 1
001 – 289128 – Jan/2016

A CIP catalogue record for this book
is available from the British Library.
ISBN 978-0-2412-4072-4

Printed and bound in Hong Kong.

All images © Dorling Kindersley Limited
For further information see: www.dkimages.com

www.dk.com

A WORLD OF IDEAS:
SEE ALL THERE IS TO KNOW

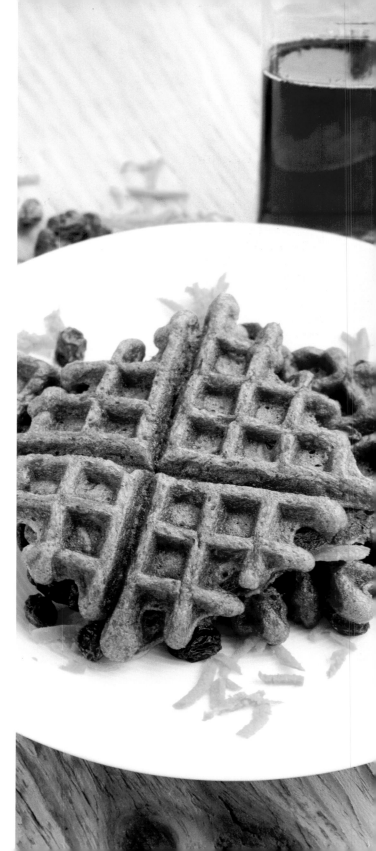

Contents

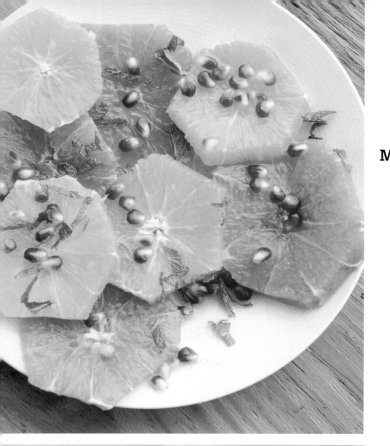

Main Courses 82

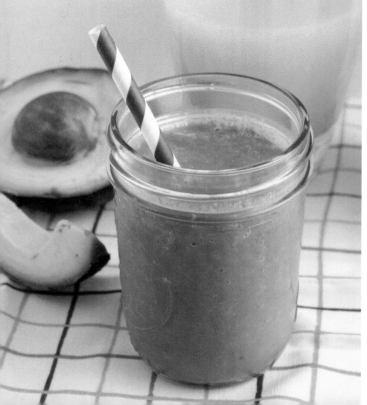

Introduction

An autoimmune disease refers to an illness characterized by a misguided immune system, which causes an attack on the body's own healthy tissues.

A common attribute of an autoimmune disorder is inflammation of the gastrointestinal system. The autoimmune protocol (AIP) diet encourages the consumption of foods that decrease inflammation, heal the gut, and assist in the restoration of healthy immune-system function.

Having worked with clients with autoimmune conditions and digestive disorders, I can appreciate and understand the challenges that come along with adopting such a unique new diet. Many fear the idea of avoiding the foods they are most familiar with. Understanding which foods to avoid and adjusting to a new way of cooking can seem daunting at first.

But take it upon yourself to channel positive creativity and curiosity. Find excitement in trying new things and experimenting with alternative ingredients. Embrace the power that comes along with being conscious of the foods you put in your body and how they make you feel.

The recipes in this book are designed to help you transition into your new AIP lifestyle without feeling deprived. In addition to delicious recipes, you will find tips and tricks to help you along the way, as well as meal plans to ensure your efforts are as successful as possible.

Acknowledgments

I would like to express my gratitude to the many people who saw me through this book. Thank you to my parents, for always believing in me and encouraging me to make my dreams a reality. From the very first day when this book was simply an idea, my family's excitement and continuous support has made this journey a memorable one. Thank you to my amazing husband, Will Thomsen, who has loved and supported me from day one when I first began experimenting in the kitchen and sharing my recipes with the world on my blog. A big thank-you to Nathalie Mornu for taking a chance on a new author and to Ann Barton, William Thomas, and the rest of the Alpha Books team for helping me bring my ideas to life. And finally, a special thanks to my registered dietician support team and friends, Jessica Bringas and Catherine Young, who tested recipes and accepted samples with open arms. I am forever grateful for my family and friends who have given me the confidence to do what I love and accomplish the unimaginable.

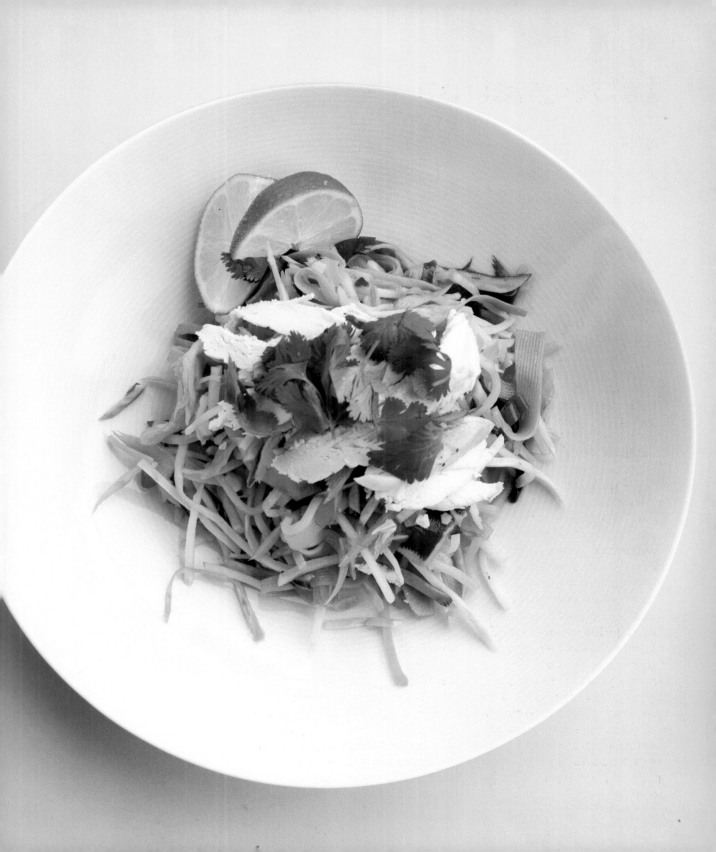

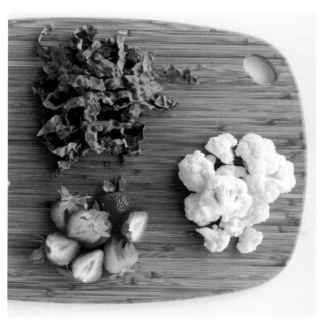
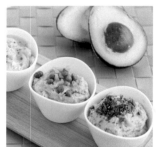
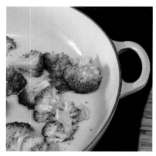

CHAPTER 1

Cooking for
HEALING

What Is **Autoimmune Disease?**

Autoimmune disease can refer to a number of illnesses that are characterized by an overactive immune system that attacks the body's healthy tissues.

Abnormal Immune Response

Disorders of the immune system cause the immune system to be abnormally underactive or overactive. In cases of immune system overactivity, such as with autoimmune disorders, the body attacks and damages its own tissues.

Antibodies are response proteins that the body produces to protect us from infection. As a defence mechanism, the body's immune system naturally produces antibodies designed to fight against foreign substances that enter the body. In the case of

autoimmune disorders, however, the immune system begins producing antibodies that attack the body's own tissues. This misdirected immune system response can lead to the destruction of healthy body tissue.

Autoimmune diseases are caused by the immune system losing the ability to differentiate proteins belonging to your own body from proteins belonging to a foreign invader (like a bacteria, virus, or parasite). Which proteins or cells are selectively attacked is what differentiates one autoimmune disease from another.

Common Autoimmune Diseases

- **Alopecia areata** Immune system attacks hair follicle cells.
- **Autoimmune hepatitis** Immune system attacks the liver.
- **Coeliac disease** Immune system attacks the lining of the small intestine.
- **Crohn's disease** Immune system attacks any part of the digestive tract, from the mouth to anus.
- **Grave's disease** Immune system attacks the thyroid, resulting in an overactive thyroid gland.
- **Hashimoto's thyroiditis** Immune system attacks the thyroid, resulting in an underactive thyroid gland.
- **Lupus** Immune system attacks cells of the skin, joints, and organs.

- **Multiple sclerosis (MS)** Immune system attacks the protective covering of nerves.
- **Pernicious anaemia** Immune system attacks cells of the stomach lining; this prevents vitamin B_{12} from being absorbed, which is critical to producing red blood cells.
- **Psoriasis** Immune system attacks skin cells.
- **Rheumatoid arthritis** Immune system attacks the joints, particularly in the hands and feet.
- **Type 1 diabetes** Immune system attacks the pancreas, resulting in the inability to produce insulin.
- **Ulcerative colitis** Immune system attacks the lining of the large intestine (colon).

Common Symptoms

The build-up of damaged cells and tissues throughout the body in an individual with an autoimmune disease can create a variety of symptoms, such as the following:

- Allergies
- Anxiety
- Digestive problems
- Extreme fatigue
- Itchy or painful skin
- Joint and muscle pain or weakness
- Low blood pressure
- Migraines or recurrent headaches
- Numbness and tingling in extremities
- Rashes
- Reduced movement and function
- Susceptibility to infection
- Swollen glands
- Thyroid problems
- Unexplained weight changes

Causes and Management

Nutrient deficiencies, genetic predisposition, accidental antibody formation, and/or leaky gut are among the triggers for an autoimmune response. Leaky gut can be brought on by infection, gut dysbiosis, dietary factors, allergies or food sensitivities, medications, chronic stress, and/or inadequate sleep. Management of an autoimmune disease generally focuses on reducing immune system activity, in part by implementing dietary protocols that assist in healing a leaky gut.

> There are more than **80 recognized autoimmune diseases,** many of which share similar symptoms, making them difficult to diagnose. Current treatments focus on **relieving symptoms** as there are no known cures.

What Is Leaky Gut?

Leaky gut refers to damage within your gastrointestinal tract that leads to gut permeability. What is gut permeability? Imagine a garden hose. When in good condition, water flows from one end of the hose to the other without leaking. If the hose becomes damaged (say we pierce the walls of the hose with a knife to create a few holes), water no longer flows seamlessly from one end to the other. Instead, due to the damage, water now leaks out of the holes. When the lining of your intestines is damaged, food no longer flows seamlessly through it. Instead, food particles leak out of the holes. However, instead of harmless water leaking out into your garden as in the hose analogy, these food participles end up in parts of your body where they don't belong. So what happens? Your immune system kicks into gear to remove these food particles so that they don't cause harm to the rest of your body. This persistent damage to the intestinal walls – commonly known as "leaky gut" – and corresponding continuous immune response is what the AIP diet is focused on repairing.

How Does **the AIP Diet** Work?

The unregulated immune system response and gut inflammation caused by autoimmune disorders can be managed with a healthy diet.

Repairing Your Gut

The autoimmune protocol (AIP) diet is a long-term health method used to address the gut inflammation that is driving an autoimmune disease. Gut inflammation causes the body to become hypersensitive to environmental triggers that an otherwise healthy person would not react to, such as certain foods.

By eliminating irritating foods that perpetuate a leaky gut and providing the body with the nourishing building blocks needed to repair the damage, this intensive healing diet allows the body to restore the balance of healthy bacteria within the gut and regulate the immune system to respond appropriately to environmental triggers, while also keeping autoimmune flare-ups at bay.

Key Nutrients

Certain vitamins and minerals support a healthy immune system and aid in decreasing inflammation throughout the body. Some of the key nutrients highlighted in the AIP diet include vitamin A, vitamin D, vitamin E, and omega-3 fatty acids.

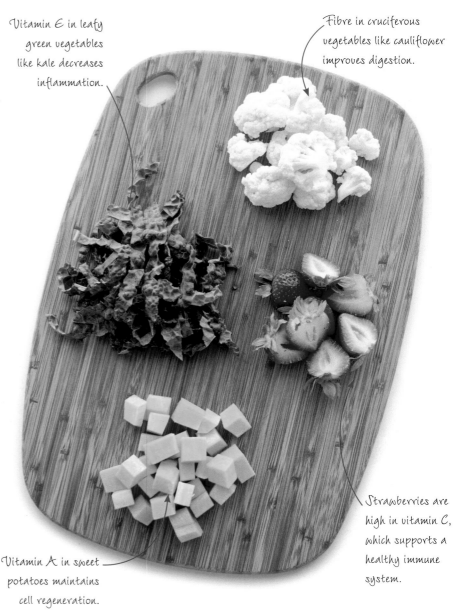

Vitamin E in leafy green vegetables like kale decreases inflammation.

Fibre in cruciferous vegetables like cauliflower improves digestion.

Strawberries are high in vitamin C, which supports a healthy immune system.

Vitamin A in sweet potatoes maintains cell regeneration.

Fuelling Your Recovery

AIP-friendly foods are those that support optimal gut health. The AIP diet eliminates foods that irritate the gut, increase gut permeability, cause gut dysbiosis (an imbalance of beneficial and harmful bacteria), or activate the immune system by causing inflammation. Examples of eliminated foods include grains, legumes, dairy, eggs, nuts, seeds, and nightshade vegetables. These foods contain compounds such as lectins and alkaloids, which are difficult for an inflamed, damaged gut to digest.

Additionally, the AIP diet encourages the consumption of foods that heal the gut, restore healthy gut bacteria, and regulate the immune system by decreasing inflammation. Examples of nutrient-dense foods rich in healing vitamins and minerals include non-nightshade vegetables, fruits, fish, quality meats, healthy fats, and probiotic-rich foods.

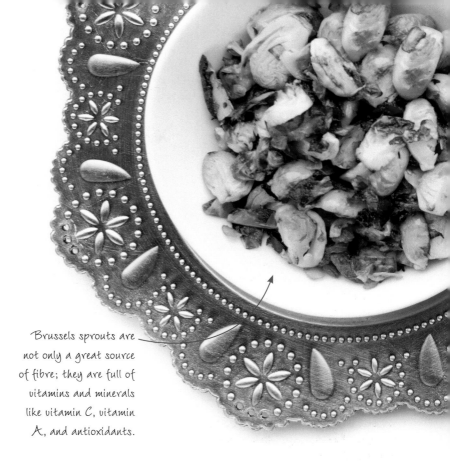

Brussels sprouts are not only a great source of fibre; they are full of vitamins and minerals like vitamin C, vitamin A, and antioxidants.

Lifestyle Factors to Support Your Diet

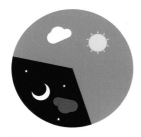

SLEEP

Giving your body time to rest is key to optimal recovery. Sleep allows your body to restore hormone levels and recharge your brain, muscles, and organs after a long day of activity and stress. Aim for at least 7 hours of sleep every night.

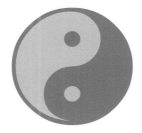

STRESS MANAGEMENT

Chronic stress can have negative consequences on the body. Whether it's taking a walk, spending time with friends, meditating, or keeping a thought journal, take steps to cope with stress in a healthy way.

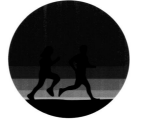

EXERCISE

Regular physical activity can have long-term health benefits and improve your quality of life. Exercise is important in managing a healthy weight, improving mood, boosting energy levels, and promoting better sleep.

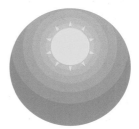

SUNLIGHT EXPOSURE

Spending time outdoors with appropriate sun exposure can increase the body's production of vitamin D. Vitamin D is important in helping the immune system function properly.

What to **Eat**

It's easy to focus on what you can't have when starting a new diet, but the AIP diet offers a robust list of delicious nutrient-dense foods to keep you satisfied.

Vegetables

- Artichoke
- Asparagus
- Beetroot
- Bok choi
- Broccoli
- Brussels sprouts
- Butternut squash
- Cabbage
- Carrot
- Cauliflower
- Celeriac/Celery root
- Celery
- Chard
- Courgette
- Cucumber
- Fennel
- Jicama
- Kale
- Leafy greens
- Leek
- Lettuce
- Mushroom
- Onion
- Parsnip
- Pumpkin
- Radish
- Rhubarb
- Salad rocket
- Shallot
- Snap peas
- Spinach
- Spring onions
- Summer squash
- Swede
- Sweet potato
- Turnip
- Watercress
- Yam

Fruits

- Apple
- Apricot
- Avocado
- Banana
- Blackberry
- Blueberry
- Cherry
- Clementine
- Coconut
- Date
- Fig
- Grape
- Grapefruit
- Guava
- Honeydew melon
- Kiwi
- Lemon
- Lime
- Mango
- Nectarine
- Orange
- Papaya
- Peach
- Pear
- Persimmon
- Plum
- Pineapple
- Pomegranate
- Raspberry
- Strawberry
- Tangerine
- Watermelon

Meat & Poultry

- Beef
- Bison
- Chicken
- Duck
- Lamb
- Offal
- Pork
- Rabbit
- Turkey
- Venison

Fish & Seafood

- Catfish
- Cod
- Clams
- Crab
- Crawfish
- Flounder
- Grouper
- Halibut
- Mussels
- Oysters
- Pollock
- Salmon
- Scallops
- Sea bass
- Shrimp
- Snapper
- Sole
- Tilapia
- Tuna

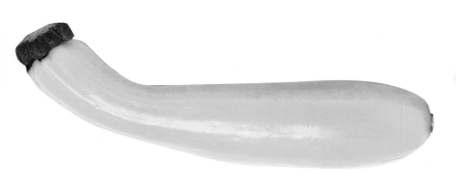
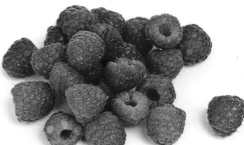

Oils & Vinegars

- Apple cider vinegar
- Balsamic vinegar
- Coconut aminos
- Coconut oil
- Olive oil
- Red wine vinegar
- Sherry vinegar
- White wine vinegar

Herbs & Spices

- Basil
- Bay leaf
- Chamomile
- Chives
- Cinnamon
- Cloves
- Coriander
- Dill
- Garlic
- Ginger
- Lavender
- Lemongrass
- Marjoram/Oregano
- Mint
- Parsley
- Peppermint
- Rosemary
- Saffron
- Sage
- Sea salt
- Spearmint
- Tarragon
- Thyme
- Turmeric

Flours & Starches

- Arrowroot powder
- Coconut flour
- Tapioca starch

Condiments & Tinned Foods

- Anchovies
- Baking soda
- Broths (vegetable, chicken, beef)
- Capers
- Coconut butter
- Coconut cream
- Coconut milk
- Fermented vegetables (pickles, sauerkraut, kimchi)
- Fish sauce
- Ghee*
- Lemon juice
- Lime juice
- Olives
- Purées (sweet potato, squash, pumpkin)
- Water chestnuts

Sweeteners

- Coconut sugar*
- Dried fruit*
- Honey*
- Maple syrup*
- Molasses*

Beverages

- Coconut water
- Coffee*
- Kombucha
- Tea (black, green, herbal)*

SOURCING INGREDIENTS

When shopping for ingredients, consider the following locations and resources for the best quality products.

Supermarket Find fresh produce, proteins, and store cupboard staples at your standard supermarkets or specialty health food store.

Farmers' Markets Get value pricing for organic produce and responsibly raised animal products at your local farmers' market.

Online Use online grocery delivery services such as Eatwild or Amazon to purchase local or hard-to-find ingredients.

* IN MODERATION

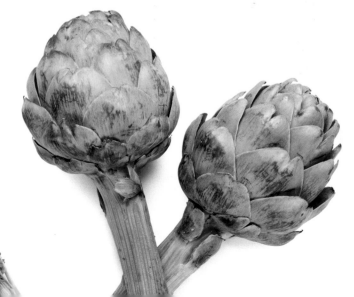

What to **Avoid**

The AIP diet eliminates foods that irritate the gut, increase gut permeability, cause gut dysbiosis, and activate the immune system by causing inflammation.

Vegetables

- Aubergine*
- Hot peppers*
- Potato*
  (varieties other than sweet potatoes)
- Sweet peppers*
- Sweetcorn
- Tomatillo*
- Tomato*

Fruits

- Goji berries*

Dairy & Eggs

- Butter
- Buttermilk
- Casein
- Cheese
- Condensed milk
- Cottage cheese
- Cream
- Cream cheese
- Eggs
- Evaporated milk
- Frozen yogurt
- Goat cheese
- Goat milk
- Ice cream
- Kefir
- Milk
- Powdered milk
- Sheep milk
- Sour cream
- Whey protein
- Whipped cream
- Yogurt

Beans & Legumes

- Adzuki beans
- Black beans
- Black-eyed beans
- Broad beans
- Butter beans
- Cannellini beans
- Chickpeas
- Kidney beans
- Lentils
- Lima beans
- Mung beans
- Navy beans
- Peanuts
- Pinto beans
- Soya beans/Edamame

Grains

- Amaranth
- Barley
- Buckwheat
- Bulgur
- Farro
- Kamut
- Millet
- Oats
- Quinoa
- Rice (all varieties)
- Rye
- Sorghum
- Spelt
- Teff
- Wheat (all varieties)

Nuts

- Almonds
- Brazil nuts
- Cashews
- Chestnuts
- Hazelnuts
- Macadamia nuts
- Pecans
- Pine nuts
- Pistachios
- Walnuts

Seeds

- Allspice
- Anise
- Caraway
- Celery seed
- Chia seeds
- Coriander
- Cumin
- Fenugreek
- Fennel seed
- Flaxseed
- Hemp seed
- Mustard seed
- Nutmeg
- Poppy seed
- Pumpkin seed
- Sesame seed
- Sunflower seed

What Are Nightshades?

Nightshades are a botanical family of plants that include tomatoes, potatoes, aubergines, and peppers. While most nightshades plants are inedible and actually poisonous, those that are edible contain compounds that make them a common food sensitivity and problematic for individuals with autoimmune diseases.

*INDICATES A NIGHTSHADE

Sweeteners

- Agave nectar
- Artificial sweeteners (acesulfame potassium, aspartame, neotame, saccharin, stevia, sucralose)
- Barley malt/Barley malt syrup
- Beetroot sugar
- Cane sugar
- Cane juice
- Corn syrup/Corn syrup solids
- Demerara sugar
- High-fructose corn syrup
- Raw sugar
- Rice syrup
- Sucanat
- Sugar alcohols (erythritol, mannitol, sorbitol, xylitol)

Oils & Vinegars

- Corn oil
- Cottonseed oil
- Hydrogenated or partially hydrogenated vegetable oil
- Palm oil
- Peanut oil
- Rapeseed oil
- Safflower oil
- Soya oil
- Sunflower oil

Other

- Alcohol
- Artificial or processed food chemicals, additives, flavourings or colouring (acrylamide, autolyzed protein, brominated vegetable oil, hydrolyzed vegetable protein, monosodium glutamate [MSG], olestra, phosphoric acid)
- Emulsifiers (carrageenan, cellulose gum, guar gum, maltodextrin, lecithin, xantham gum)
- Herbs/Spices (ashwaganda, cayenne pepper*, chilli pepper flakes*, chilli powder*, curry powder, paprika*)
- Soya (seitan, soya lecithin, soy sauce, tamari, tempeh, textured vegetable protein, tofu)
- Yeast

INFLAMMATORY COMPOUNDS

Many eliminated foods on the AIP diet contain the following compounds, which are difficult for an inflamed, damaged gut to digest and inhibit beneficial gut healing and restoration of healthy gut bacteria.

Lectins These sugar-binding proteins found in nightshades protect plants from predation. The compounds are resistant to digestion, inflammatory, and have the ability to increase intestinal permeability.

Alkaloids These compounds found in nightshades can contribute to gut irritation and leaky gut.

Solanine This compound gives potatoes their bitter taste.

Capsaicin This compound gives peppers their heat.

Cooking with Alcohol

Some recipes in this book include wine or Cognac to enhance the flavour of the finished dish. While alcohol is on the list of foods to avoid, cooking with wine or spirits over high heat allows for most of the damaging alcohol to cook off before the final product ever reaches your plate.

Stocking Your Store Cupboard
with Staples

Keeping your kitchen stocked with the following pantry staples
will make cooking AIP-friendly recipes a breeze.

Anchovies
These small fish are great for adding
flavour to dressings, sauces, and salads.

Arrowroot powder
This starch can be used in baked goods
or as a thickening agent.

Baking powder
Baking powder may contain cornflour, so
instead of 1 tsp. baking powder, use
½ tsp. bicarbonate of soda mixed with ¼
tsp. cream of tartar.

Bicarbonate of soda
This fine white powder acts as a leavening
agent in baked goods.

Balsamic vinegar
Made from wine vinegar blended with
grape juice, the traditional sweet-and-sour
taste makes this vinegar perfect for salad
dressings, sauces, and cooked meats.

Canned seafood
Keep canned tuna, salmon, sardines,
oysters, and herring on hand for a quick
lunch or snack.

Capers
The edible flower bud of the caper plant is
salted and pickled for use as a culinary
seasoning or garnish. Capers are used in
sauces, meat dishes, and salads.

Carob powder
This sweet edible pulp comes from a pod
of the Mediterranean carob tree. The pulp
is dried and roasted into a caffeine-free
smooth powder, which can be substituted
for cocoa powder in nearly every recipe.

Cider vinegar
Made from apples, this vinegar is high in
acetic acid, which has potent
antimicrobial properties.

Coconut aminos
Coconut aminos is a soya-free seasoning
(similar in flavour to soy sauce) that is
made by fermenting coconut tree sap.

Coconut butter
Coconut butter is a thick and smooth butter
made from the flesh of the coconut. It is
thicker and richer than coconut oil.

Coconut flour
This soft, dense flour comes from dried,
ground coconut meat and can be used in
baking. Because it is so absorbent, you only
need to substitute 25g (scant 1oz) coconut
flour for every 100g (3½ oz) regular flour.

Coconut milk and cream
Coconut milk and cream are made by
combining shredded coconut with water.
Coconut cream is thicker and richer in
flavour than coconut milk.

Coconut

You may have noticed the prevalence of coconut
products that fit within the AIP diet. The versatile fruit
of the coconut tree is the basis for many AIP-friendly
products that can stand in for
a variety of off-limits foods,
including conventional flour
and sugar, dairy products,
and soy sauce.

Coconut oil

Coconut oil is extracted from coconut meat. This oil contains lauric acid, an easily digestible, antimicrobial fat that helps reduce inflammation. Look for unrefined virgin or pure coconut oil that has not been bleached or deodorized.

Coconut sugar

Coconut sugar is produced from the liquid sap of cut flower buds of the coconut palm tree.

Dried fruit

Keep dried fruits like raisins, dates, prunes, and apricots on hand for sweeteners in recipes or for a quick snack.

Fish sauce

Known for its savoury, sweet, and umani flavours, fish sauce is extracted from fermented anchovies. Look for brands that do not contain any additional preservatives or monosodium glutamate.

Gelatine

Typically found in powder form, gelatine is derived from the collagen of animal by-products (skin, tendons, ligaments, and bones) and is commonly used in the production of jellies. It can be used as a binder in cooking or taken as a supplement to support joint health.

Ghee

Ghee, also referred to as clarified butter, is made by heating butter to separate and remove the milk solids which contain lactose and milk proteins. Ghee can be made at home or purchased commercially.

Honey

Honey can be used to sweeten dressings and desserts. Choose organic raw, unfiltered honey.

Fermented Foods

Fermented foods contain naturally occurring beneficial probiotics and digestive enzymes that help boost the immune system and support a healthy gut. Whether you enjoy kombucha, pickles, or sauerkraut, read the ingredient label closely to ensure the product doesn't contain nightshades.

Lemon and lime juice

Purchasing pre-squeezed fresh lemon and lime juices for use in dressings and sauces will save you time when it comes to food preparation.

Maple syrup

Maple syrup can be used to sweeten dressing and desserts. Try Grade B maple syrup, which has a strong maple flavour and sweet caramel undertones.

Molasses

Molasses can be used to sweeten sauces and baked goods. With its dark colour and thick consistency, blackstrap molasses has a rich flavour and superior mineral content.

Olive oil

Olive oil is a great source of healthy monounsaturated fats. Look for virgin or extra-virgin varieties.

Olives

Olives are an easy way to add flavour to a salad or meal.

Purées

Canned sweet potato, squash, and pumpkin purées can save you time in the kitchen. Use purées to thicken soups or to create a quick side dish in a pinch.

Red wine vinegar

Red wine vinegar is made from fermented and aged diluted red wine. Red wine vinegar is great for salad dressings, sauces, and pickling.

Sherry vinegar

Sherry vinegar is made from fermented sherry and adds a gourmet flavour to any vinaigrette.

Stocks

Keep your pantry and freezer stocked with vegetable, chicken, and beef stock for use in soups and stews. When purchasing stocks, read the ingredients to ensure there are no artificial flavours or additives.

Tapioca starch

Extracted from the cassava plant, this starchy white flour can be used in baked goods or as a thickening agent.

Water chestnuts

This starchy aquatic vegetable is typically found in a can and is commonly used in Asian cuisines. Its fresh taste and crunchy texture are a perfect addition to sautéed veggies or stir-fries.

White wine vinegar

White wine vinegar is made from fermented and aged diluted white wine.

Making Good **Food Choices**

Even working within the AIP guidelines, it's easy to feel overwhelmed by the options available at your supermarket.

Reading Food Labels

Informed food choices begins with understanding food labelling. The more information you can learn about a product, the better. Look for verification symbols and review the list of ingredients. Ingredients are listed in order of dominance, so the most prevalent ingredients are listed first. Look for products with short lists of ingredients and words you recognize. If you can't pronounce an ingredient or have questions about the quality and sourcing of the product, avoid it.

Natural
Should refer to single foods to which nothing has been added and which have been subjected only to traditional processing, such as smoking, drying, or fermentation. However, regulations for this term are more lenient than for organic labelling and "natural" products may still contain antibiotics and growth hormones.

Pure
Refers to single foods or a food in the ingredients (e.g. "pure-butter shortbread") to show that the ingredients have not been mixed with others.

Free-Range
Refers to animals that are allowed access to the outdoors; however, the quality and size of the outdoor space, and the duration of time allotted to animals to roam outdoors, may not be regulated. Remember, organic always means free-range in the purest sense of the term, but free-range by itself never means organic systems are in place.

Sustainable Seafood
Refers to seafood that is either caught or farmed in a way that considers the well-being of the harvested species as well as its surrounding environment.

Organic
According to EU regulations, organic plants must be grown without conventional pesticides, synthetic fertilizers, sewage sludge, genetically modified ingredients, or ionizing radiation. Organic meat and poultry must come from animals that are given no antibiotics or growth hormones. Look out for the Soil Association's Organic Standard logo, which can be found on around 80 per cent of organic produce in the UK.

Buying Organic
The Dirty Dozen list refers to conventional, non-organic fruits and vegetables that contain the highest amount of pesticide residues. Fruits and vegetables on the Clean Fifteen list contain the fewest pesticides. When shopping for organics, prioritize items on the AIP Dirty Dozen list.

THE AIP DIRTY DOZEN

Apples	Kale
Berries	Nectarines
Celery	Peaches
Cucumbers	Peas
Grapes	Spinach
Greens	Courgettes

THE AIP CLEAN FIFTEEN

Asparagus	Kiwi fruits
Avocados	Mangos
Cabbages	Mushrooms
Cantaloupes	Onions
Cauliflower	Papayas
Citrus (lemon, lime, orange, grapefruit)	Pineapples
	Sweet potatoes
Honeydew melons	Watermelons

AIP Food Choice Guide

	GOOD	BETTER	BEST
FRUITS AND VEGETABLES	Conventional fruits and vegetables	Utilizing the AIP Dirty Dozen and AIP Clean Fifteen lists	All organic, local, and seasonal produce
MEAT AND POULTRY	Antibiotic-free and hormone-free	Grass-fed and/or organic	Organic, and pasture-raised
SEAFOOD	Farm-raised seafood	Canned or frozen wild-caught seafood	Fresh, local, and sustainably wild-caught seafood
FATS	Conventional grain-fed ghee	Organic ghee, conventional coconut oil, conventional olive oil	Organic lard, tallow, or ghee; organic extra-virgin coconut or olive oil
SWEETENERS	Unrefined cane sugar	Coconut sugar, conventional honey, or maple syrup	Raw organic honey, organic real maple syrup

Making the Most of Your **Budget**

Eating healthy doesn't have to be expensive. Practise buying in bulk, shopping seasonally, and repurposing leftovers to make the most of your food purchases.

Buying in Bulk

The goal of buying in bulk is to reduce waste and save money. When done right, this method of shopping can yield big returns on the investment in the form of time and money.

Bulk Bins

More and more supermarkets and health-food stores are offering customers the ability to buy produce by weight. Often stored in large "bulk bins", items on offer can include a variety of items such as dried spices, dried mushrooms, dried fruit, coconut flour, arrowroot powder, tapioca starch, loose teas, olive oil, vinegars, honey, and maple syrup.

Less Packaging = Money Saved

Items purchased in bulk are sold without packaging, meaning one less step for the manufacturer. This decreases the overall cost of the goods. Less packaging also means less waste and therefore a smarter environmental choice.

Price per Unit

Not all items can be purchased loose by weight. For items purchased frequently, look for larger packages. Check the unit price on your favourite grocery items; you will most likely notice that items purchased in a larger size or quantity typically cost less per unit than their smaller counterparts. Some supermarkets even offer discounts if purchasing items in cases. Depending on your kitchen storage space, stock up on pantry staples like stocks, coconut milk, and canned fish to save time and money.

Buy Only What You Need

Bulk bins allow you to purchase only what you need. Whether it's 1 kilogram or 1 teaspoon, you can avoid wasting product by scaling your purchase to the amount needed at the time of purchase.

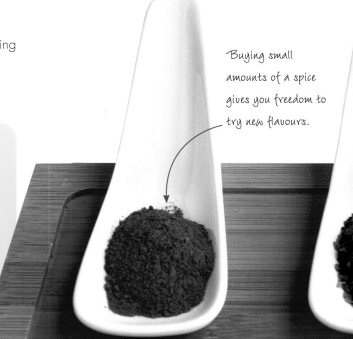

Buying small amounts of a spice gives you freedom to try new flavours.

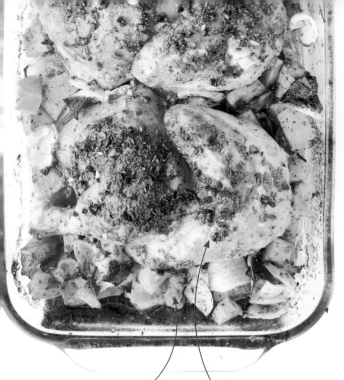

Swap sweet potatoes for summer squash, depending on the season.

Freeze individual servings of leftover chicken for quick additions to soups and salads.

Use a clean scoop to help avoid cross-contamination.

Shopping Locally and Seasonally

Local food refers to food that is grown or raised and harvested close to the consumers' homes. Because of this close proximity, the food is distributed over a much shorter distance than is common in the conventional global industrial food system. Most crops are picked at the peak of ripeness and transported directly to a market or farm shop. Therefore, local food systems are generally associated with higher-quality ingredients at a lower cost. Shopping locally also allows you the opportunity to develop a personal relationship with the farmer or food processor. Ask questions about how the food is grown or raised, what sustainability measures are being executed, and details about quality control. Shopping seasonally is also important when looking for value. Purchasing foods that are in season in your area will yield the best-tasting food at the lowest cost.

Plan Ahead and Repurpose Leftovers

When batch-cooking or buying in bulk, it's important to think about how these items will be used. Make time to plan how you'll use these foods in recipes and meals. For example, leftover **Greek-Style Roast Chicken** can be repurposed for making Avocado Chicken Salad or Classic Chicken and Cauliflower Soup.

Beware of Cross-Contamination

If your supermarket also sells items on the **Foods to Avoid** list in the bulk bins, be cautious. Scoops used for gluten-containing foods or nuts and seeds could potentially end up in bins where they don't belong. If the bulk department where you shop doesn't appear to be taking active measures to avoid cross-contamination, you may be better off hitting the aisles for prepackaged goods instead to decrease your chances of unintentional exposure to inflammatory foods.

Saving Time in the Kitchen

Following an AIP diet doesn't have to mean cooking every day. With planning and preparation, you can make the most of your time and ingredients.

Batch Cooking

Batch cooking refers to preparing meals and snacks ahead of time to be eaten in the future. For example, this could mean cooking one day to prepare most or all of your meals and snacks to be eaten for the entire week ahead. By spending a few hours in your kitchen during one day a week, you can save yourself the headache of deciding what to make for dinner and the time of cooking everything from scratch during the week. Focus on completing the hard parts of food preparation early on to set yourself up for success when life gets busy. Batch cooking saves you time and allows you to enjoy time with loved ones, take interest in new hobbies, exercise, meditate, or decompress guilt-free, knowing that you have fuelled your body optimally.

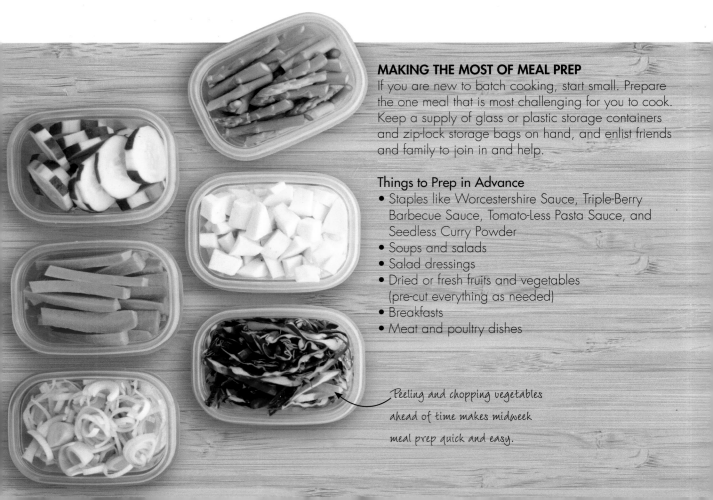

MAKING THE MOST OF MEAL PREP

If you are new to batch cooking, start small. Prepare the one meal that is most challenging for you to cook. Keep a supply of glass or plastic storage containers and zip-lock storage bags on hand, and enlist friends and family to join in and help.

Things to Prep in Advance
- Staples like Worcestershire Sauce, Triple-Berry Barbecue Sauce, Tomato-Less Pasta Sauce, and Seedless Curry Powder
- Soups and salads
- Salad dressings
- Dried or fresh fruits and vegetables (pre-cut everything as needed)
- Breakfasts
- Meat and poultry dishes

Peeling and chopping vegetables ahead of time makes midweek meal prep quick and easy.

Meal Planning

Treat your meal plan like you would any other appointment or meeting in your life. You wouldn't skip a meeting with your boss, so why miss a date with your dinner plans? Plan what you are going to eat for the week and stick to it. Use the Weekly Meal Plans and Shopping Lists to help get you started. Create your own meal plan by using the tips below.

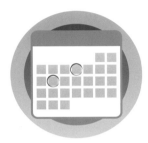

Look at your schedule.
Based on your current life commitments, determine the days and time you can commit to cooking. If you're going to be home late, plan a slow-cooker meal so that the cooking can be done when you walk through the door. Knowing your schedule for the week ahead leaves little room for surprises and excuses.

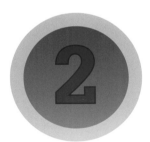

Choose ONE item for breakfast.
Buy enough ingredients for all seven days of the week and batch cook as needed on the weekend. Whether you make individual servings of Crisp Ham Cups or a batch of Apple Cinnamon Hearts Cereal, make enough to cover every morning of your week.

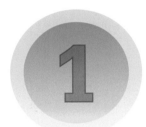

Choose TWO items to make for lunches.
Select two soup or salad recipes to use for lunches throughout the week. Make sure you have plenty of glass or plastic containers and zip-lock bags available for packing things like dressings and salad toppings.

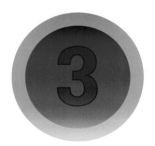

Choose THREE dinner meal ideas for dinner.
Select 3 of your favourite dinner recipes to make for dinner throughout the week. Refer to the section on Batch Cooking to help guide you in preparing ahead of time and minimize time spent in the kitchen during a busy week.

Kitchen **Tools & Equipment**

Most of what you need to cook for an AIP diet is probably already in your kitchen. Here are some specific tools that are used throughout the book.

Special Tools

Blender
A high-speed blender with a strong motor is a great investment when cooking for an AIP lifestyle. Invest in brands like Vitamix, BlendTec, and Breville and look for a model with a tamper accessory that allows you to push contents toward the blade while blending.

Electric mixer
Electric mixers come in all shapes and sizes. Either a stand mixer or an inexpensive hand mixer can be used for the recipes in this book.

Food processor
Choose a mid-sized (1.5–2 litres/ 2¾–3½ pints) food processor with basic slicer and shredder discs to make everything from smooth purées to perfectly shredded slaws.

Grill pan
Grill pans are great for indoor grilling all year long. Choose a ridged grill pan that is heavy-duty aluminium, stainless steel, or cast iron for consistent and even cooking. The ridges hold food up and away from the fat and juices that are rendered during cooking.

Ice lolly mould
Plastic ice lolly moulds are generally sold in sets of six ice lollies and are an easy way to make your favourite frozen treats.

Juicer
Juicing is a great way to obtain a large amount of nutrients in a small volume. Select a juicer that is easy to clean with pieces that are dishwasher safe.

Mandolin
Choose a mandolin with a variety of blades to create uniform slices and juliennes. Look for an easily adjustable blade for creating a variety of thicknesses and a basic hand guard for safety.

Meat thermometer
A meat thermometer is a lifesaver for the novice cook. Select an inexpensive digital meat thermometer and keep extra batteries on hand to ensure you know when your meat is done at all times.

Mesh sieve
A mesh sieve is handy for draining steamed vegetables or straining homemade bone broths and stocks.

 BLENDER   **ELECTRIC MIXER**   **FOOD PROCESSOR**   **GRILL OR GRILL PAN**   **ICE LOLLY MOULDS**   **JUICE**   **MANDOLIN**   **MEAT THERMOMETER**   **MESH SIEVE**

MORTAR & PESTLE **MUFFIN TIN** **OVEN-PROOF FRYING PAN** **SLOW COOKER** **SPIRALIZER** **STOCK POT OR DUTCH OVEN** **WAFFLE IRON** **WOODEN SKEWERS**

Mortar and pestle

A mortar and pestle comes in handy for grinding up spices quickly and easily. However, an electric spice grinder is preferred for tougher-to-handle spices.

Muffin tin

While baked goods like muffins don't appear frequently on the AIP diet, a muffin tin is great for making individual-portioned entrées such as mini meatloaves.

Ovenproof frying pan

A frying pan with sloped slides that is larger than a traditional frying pan. An ovenproof frying pan with a tight-fitting lid is most versatile.

Slow cooker

A slow cooker is an indispensable appliance for anyone with a busy lifestyle. Choose a size that is compatible with your household; a 3½–4 litre (6¼–7 pints) size typically feeds a family of four, while a 5–6 litre (8¾–10½ pints) size is better for larger households. Programmable slow cookers that automatically switch to warm after the cooking time is complete are crucial for anyone with an unpredictable schedule.

Spiralizer

A spiralizer is an inexpensive and fun kitchen tool to have on hand to make fresh veggie noodles. Look for a spiralizer with a variety of blades to make noodles of all shapes and sizes.

Stock pot or Dutch oven

A large stock pot is key for making batches of soups and stews. Even better, the versatility of a Dutch oven with a tight-fitting lid allows it to be used on the hob and be transferred to the oven with ease.

Waffle iron

An waffle iron is great for making breakfast on special occasions. Save space in the kitchen by opting for a smaller, inexpensive one for easy storage; you can always cook in batches when company visits.

Wooden skewers

Use wooden skewers for kebabs and grilling. Thread your favourite meat and veggies onto moist kebabs and put on the grill for a quick dinner.

OTHER USEFUL TOOLS AND APPLIANCES

Baking tins
Baking sheets & trays
Baster
Basting brush
Chef's knife
Colander
Cutting boards
Dehydrator
Kitchen scissors

Ladle
Measuring jugs
Measuring spoons
Meat tenderizer
Mixing bowls (small, medium, and large)
Peeler
Plastic squeeze bottles
Preserving jars
Salad spinner

Saucepans
Sealable containers
Slotted spoon
Spatula
Tin opener
Tongs
Whisk
Wooden spoons
Zester

Ensuring Success

Adapting the AIP diet takes time. Understanding foods to avoid and adjusting to new ways of cooking can seem daunting at first. Keep these tips in mind to ensure your transition to an AIP-friendly lifestyle is as successful as possible.

Top 5 Ways to Avoid Temptation

1 Clean Out Your Store Cupboard
Recruit your entire household to support you in your new AIP-friendly lifestyle. Remove all items from your freezer, fridge, and pantry that are on the **What to Avoid** food list. Non-AIP foods brought into the house by family and friends only create temptations. Keep your kitchen stocked with foods on the **What to Eat** list and leave all foods on the **What to Avoid** list on the supermarket shelves.

2 Love Your Leftovers
Temptation can strike at any time. Maybe you have a late night at the office, are unable to spend time on the weekend batch cooking due to busy family schedules, or you come home from vacation to an empty fridge. Whatever the situation is, leftovers can come in handy when managing a busy lifestyle. You can never have too many extra meals for unexpected situations. Make extra today and you will thank yourself tomorrow – or three months from now.

3 Create New Habits
If you previously ordered pizza on weekend nights or Chinese takeaway every Wednesday, it's time to form new habits to avoid feeling deprived. Following an AIP diet is easier if you cook at home since you will have control over each and every ingredient within the meal. Find joy in batch cooking on the weekends and start new traditions like Soup Sundays, Slow Cooker Saturdays, or Fish Fridays.

4 Find AIP-friendly Substitutions
When sweet or salty cravings strike, be prepared. Avoid reaching for non-AIP-approved foods when temptation surfaces by stocking your kitchen with ready-to-eat snacks and treats.

5 Cook for Your Family and Friends
Embrace the curiosity of your loved ones. Educate them on your new style of eating and surprise them with a delicious AIP-friendly dinner party.

Expand Your Palate

While some familiar ingredients may be off-limits, supermarkets offer more variety than ever. Take advantage of new, unfamiliar ingredients and don't be afraid of something new—you never know what foods might become your new favourites! The following are some of the less-familiar fruits and vegetables you can expect to try throughout this cookbook.

- Butternut squash
- Fennel
- Ginger
- Kale
- Leeks
- Parsnips
- Pomegranate
- Portobello mushrooms
- Spaghetti squash
- Swedes

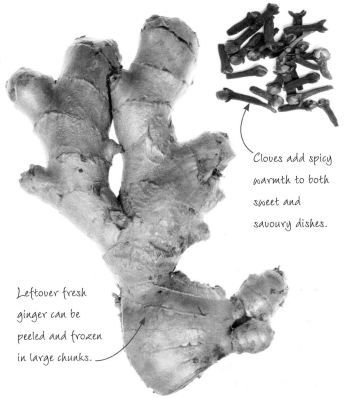

Cloves add spicy warmth to both sweet and savoury dishes.

Leftover fresh ginger can be peeled and frozen in large chunks.

The Importance of Herbs and Spices

Don't just rely on salt to flavour your food. Spices and herbs add flavour, warmth, and depth to your basic ingredients and can affect the whole flavour profile of a dish. Use turmeric or ginger for an Asian-inspired cuisine. Rely on oregano and basil for an Italian twist, or garlic and fresh coriander for Mexican flavours.

Words of Encouragement

Start slow
Adopting an AIP lifestyle doesn't happen overnight and it's easy to become overwhelmed. Start slow and take small steps. Understanding and implementing the AIP diet is a learning process.

Embrace mistakes
Forming new eating habits is challenging. Mistakes are inevitable. Strive for progress, not perfection.

Seek support
Nothing is more powerful than a network of support. Encourage your friends and family to try new recipes with you. Join community groups and online forums to meet individuals experiencing the same struggles.

Practise with patience
The more AIP-friendly meals you are familiar with, the easier eating and cooking for your unique condition will become. Continued practice in the kitchen will make your new eating habits second nature.

Be prepared
You can't always predict your next meal. Whether you keep a few frozen AIP-friendly meals in the office freezer or pack dried fruit in the glove box of your car for an emergency snack, it's always better to be overly prepared.

Staple Recipes

Avoid added sugars and unwanted spices by making your own pantry staples from scratch.

There are many basic pantry staples we rely on to cook delicious meals. However, some of these items contain ingredients that are not AIP-friendly, such as sugar, artificial flavourings, and spices derived from seeds.

Many recipes throughout this book rely on the following staple recipes for key ingredients, which appear in bold on the ingredients list.

- Bone Broth
- Basic Avocado "Mayonnaise"
- Worcestershire Sauce
- Triple-Berry Barbecue Sauce
- Tomato-Less Pasta Sauce
- Seed-Free Curry Powder

Stock Up on Staples

Save the bones from chicken, pork, and beef meals and keep a continuous collection in a zipper-lock plastic bag in the freezer until you have enough bones to make a batch of **Bone Broth**. Freeze broth in small batches or in an ice-cube tray so you have easy access to the necessary portion sizes when needed.

Make several batches of **Seed-Free Curry Powder** and store it in an airtight jar in the pantry.

Freeze **Basic Avocado "Mayonnaise"** in small batches using an ice-cube tray. Thaw in the fridge overnight when ready to use.

Prepare a few batches of **Triple-Berry Barbecue Sauce** and **Tomato-Less Pasta Sauce** and freeze them in small containers for use as needed.

Worcestershire Sauce can be made ahead and kept in the refrigerator for up to one month.

This **mineral-rich savoury broth** can be used as a base for soups or stews, or consumed as a beverage for a quick nutritious boost.

Bone Broth

 YIELD: **1.5 LITRES (2¾ PINTS)** SERVING SIZE: **240ML (8 FL OZ)** PREP TIME: **5 MINUTES** COOK TIME: **24 HOURS**

INGREDIENTS

2 roasted chicken carcasses (about 680g [1½ lbs.] of bones)

2 stalks celery, chopped into large chunks

2 carrots, unpeeled and chopped into large chunks

1 medium yellow onion, unpeeled and quartered

1 head garlic, sliced, unpeeled and halved lengthwise

1 bay leaf

5–10 sprigs fresh thyme

5–10 sprigs fresh parsley

2 tbsp cider vinegar

1.5 litres (2¾ pints) water

Salt

SPECIAL TOOLS

 SLOW COOKER

 FINE MESH SIEVE

METHOD

1 Put bones, celery, and carrots in a slow cooker. Add onion, garlic, bay leaf, thyme, and parsley.

2 Add cider vinegar and enough water to cover all of the bones and vegetables. Cook on low for 24 hours.

3 Using a slotted spoon, remove and discard the vegetables and bones.

4 Using a fine mesh sieve, strain the broth into a large container or several small containers. Cover and refrigerate overnight or until chilled.

5 Scrape fat from the top of the broth and discard. Taste and season with salt as needed.

Storage: After removing the fat layer from the broth, store in the refrigerator for up to 1 week or freeze for up to 6 months.

You can use any mix of beef, pork, or chicken bones for making bone broth. Adding meaty bones such as short ribs or ham bones will add extra flavour to your broth.

NUTRITION

Calories **86**

Total Fat **3g**

Saturated Fat **1g**

Unsaturated Fat **2g**

Cholesterol **7mg**

Sodium **45mg**

Carbohydrate **0g**

Dietary Fibre **0g**

Sugar **0g**

Protein **6g**

In this versatile recipe, tart cider vinegar and lemon juice accompany the **creamy texture of the avocado** to create the perfect mayonnaise substitute.

Basic **Avocado "Mayonnaise"**

 YIELD: **240ML**   SERVING SIZE: **2 TBSP**   PREP TIME: **10 MINUTES**   COOK TIME: **NONE**

INGREDIENTS

1 medium avocado

2 tbsp cider vinegar

2 tbsp olive oil

2¼ tsp lemon juice

½ tsp salt

SPECIAL TOOLS

 FOOD PROCESSOR

METHOD

1 Cut avocado in half and discard the pit. Scoop avocado flesh from skin and place in a food processor.

2 Add cider vinegar, olive oil, lemon juice, and salt. Process for 30 seconds or until smooth.

Storage: Store in an airtight container for up to 3 days or freeze in an ice-cube tray for single serving use for up to 3 months.

Serving suggestion: Dip Rosemary Sweet Potato Chips into Garlic Herb Mayo or drizzle Wasabi Avocado Mayo over Honey Ginger Glazed Salmon.

Variations: For **Garlic Herb Avocado Mayo,** add 2 garlic cloves, 2 tbsp fresh parsley, 2 tbsp fresh rosemary, and 2 tbsp fresh thyme.

For **Wasabi Avocado Mayo,** add 2 tsp wasabi powder and 1½ tsp coconut aminos.

For **Tartar Sauce Mayo,** substitute cider vinegar for white wine vinegar and add 70g (2½ oz) chopped dill pickles, 2 tbsp capers, and ¼ tsp fresh horseradish.

Use this AIP-friendly mayo for any recipe that calls for regular mayo to avoid processed oils, eggs, and dairy.

NUTRITION

Calories **76**

Total Fat **8g**

Saturated Fat **1g**

Unsaturated Fat **6g**

Cholesterol **0mg**

Sodium **147mg**

Carbohydrate **3g**

Dietary Fibre **2g**

Sugar **0g**

Protein **1g**

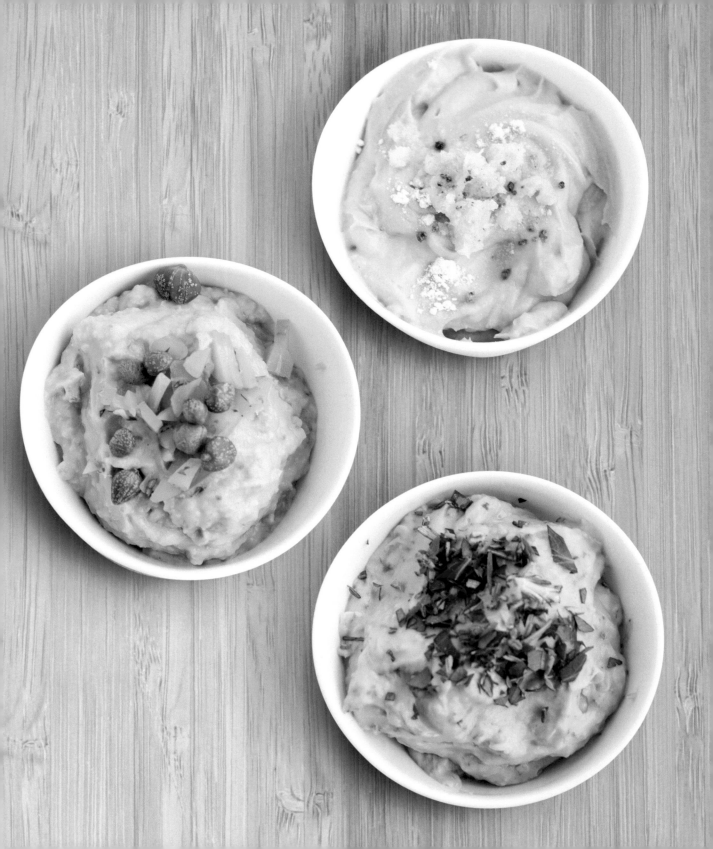

Like the bought version, this quick and easy sauce is **bursting with bold, sweet, sour, and salty flavours**, but it uses only AIP-friendly ingredients.

Worcestershire Sauce

 YIELD: **125ML**   SERVING SIZE: **1 TSP**   PREP TIME: **3 MINUTES**   COOK TIME: **NONE**

INGREDIENTS

125ml (4fl oz) cider vinegar

2 tbsp fish sauce

1 tbsp honey

1 tbsp molasses

1 tbsp lime juice

¼ tsp ground cloves

¼ tsp garlic powder

½ tsp onion powder

SPECIAL TOOLS

 BLENDER

METHOD

1 In a blender or food processor, combine cider vinegar, fish sauce, honey, molasses, lime juice, ground cloves, garlic powder, and onion powder.

2 Process for 30 seconds or until smooth and combined.

Storage: Store in an airtight container in the fridge for up to 1 month.

Fish sauce is an umami-rich flavouring agent extracted from salted and fermented anchovies. Be sure to select a brand without added sugar.

NUTRITION

Calories **7**	Saturated Fat **0g**	Cholesterol **0g**	Carbohydrate **2g**	Sugar **1g**
Total Fat **0g**	Unsaturated Fat **0g**	Sodium **125g**	Dietary Fibre **0g**	Protein **0g**

This **smoky and sweet barbecue sauce** is completely nightshade free. Bacon fat and Worcestershire Sauce add depth and tangy flavour.

Triple-Berry **Barbecue Sauce**

 YIELD: 450ML   **SERVING SIZE: 50ml**   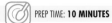 **PREP TIME: 10 MINUTES**   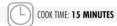 **COOK TIME: 15 MINUTES**

INGREDIENTS

1 tbsp bacon fat

300g (10½oz) onion, chopped (1 large onion)

150g (5½oz) carrots, peeled and chopped (2 large carrots)

3 cloves garlic, finely chopped

66g (2½oz) strawberries, chopped

70g (2½oz) cherries, pitted

35g (1¼oz) blueberries

50ml (2fl oz) maple syrup

3 tbsp Worcestershire Sauce

1 tbsp apple cider vinegar

2 tbsp coconut aminos

2 tbsp molasses

125ml (4fl oz) beef stock

½ tsp smoked sea salt

SPECIAL TOOLS

 BLENDER

METHOD

1 In a medium saucepan, combine bacon fat, onion, carrots, and garlic. Cook for 5 minutes over a medium-high heat or until vegetables begin to soften.

2 Add strawberries, cherries, blueberries, maple syrup, Worcestershire Sauce, cider vinegar, coconut aminos, molasses, beef stock, and smoked sea salt.

3 Stir to combine and bring contents to the boil. Reduce heat and simmer for 10 minutes.

4 Transfer contents to a high-speed blender and blend until smooth.

Storage: Store sauce in an airtight jar or squeeze bottle for up to 2 weeks.

Serving suggestion: Use with Triple-Berry Barbecue Ribs or New Orleans Barbecue Shrimp, or mix into Orange Pulled Pork Carnitas for an easy barbecue pulled pork.

NUTRITION

| Calories 109 | Saturated Fat 1g | Cholesterol 2g | Carbohydrate 23g | Sugar 16g |
| Total Fat 2g | Unsaturated Fat 1g | Sodium 114g | Dietary Fibre 2g | Protein 1g |

With red beetroot, creamy sweet potatoes, and savoury onion and garlic, this **tomato-free sauce has all of the flavours you love,** without the nightshades.

Tomato-Less **Pasta Sauce**

 YIELD: **450ML**   SERVING SIZE: **125ML**   PREP TIME: **10 MINUTES**   COOK TIME: **20 MINUTES**

INGREDIENTS

2 tbsp olive oil

300g (10½ oz) onion, chopped (1 large onion)

4 garlic cloves, minced

150g (5½ oz) carrot, chopped

110g (4oz) celery, chopped

1 tbsp beetroot, peeled and finely chopped

1 tbsp balsamic vinegar

4 tsp lemon juice

2 tbsp sweet potato purée

1 tsp dried basil

1 tsp dried thyme

1 tsp dried oregano

½ tsp salt

450ml (16fl oz) vegetable stock

SPECIAL TOOLS

 BLENDER

METHOD

1 Heat a large saucepan over a medium-high heat. Add oil, onion, garlic, carrot, celery, and beetroot. Sauté for 5 minutes or until the vegetables begin to soften.

2 Add balsamic vinegar, lemon juice, sweet potato purée, ½ tsp basil, ½ tsp thyme, ½ tsp oregano, salt, and vegetable stock.

3 Bring sauce to the boil, reduce heat, and cover. Simmer for 10 minutes.

4 Remove pan from heat. In a high-speed blender, blend sauce until smooth.

5 Return sauce to pan and add remaining ½ tsp basil, ½ tsp thyme, and ½ tsp oregano.

Storage: Store sauce in an airtight container in the fridge for 1 week or freeze for up to 3 months.

Serving Suggestion: Serve sauce over Herbed-Baked Spaghetti Squash for a quick dinner, or add to your favourite soup or stew recipe for a burst of umami flavour.

NUTRITION

Calories **132**

Total Fat **7g**

Saturated Fat **1g**

Unsaturated Fat **6g**

Cholesterol **0mg**

Sodium **619mg**

Carbohydrate **16g**

Dietary Fibre **3g**

Sugar **7g**

Protein **2g**

Like traditional curry powders, this **curry powder alternative** is savory and robust. It will add a **bold, spicy flavour** to almost any dish.

Seed-Free **Curry Powder**

 YIELD: **2½ TBSP** SERVING SIZE: **1½ TSP** PREP TIME: **3 MINUTES** COOK TIME: **NONE**

INGREDIENTS

1½ tsp onion powder

1½ tsp garlic powder

1½ tsp dried turmeric

1 tsp dried coriander

1 tsp dried basil

½ tsp dried dill

½ tsp ground cinnamon

½ tsp ground ginger

¼ tsp ground cloves

METHOD

1 In a mortar and pestle or spice grinder, combine onion powder, garlic powder, turmeric, coriander, basil, dill, cinnamon, ginger, and cloves.

2 Grind to a fine powder. Once you have reached the desired consistency, transfer to an airtight container.

Storage: Store in an airtight container away from heat and light for up to 6 months.

SPECIAL TOOLS

 MORTAR AND PESTLE

NUTRITION

Calories **10**

Total Fat **0g**

Saturated Fat **0g**

Unsaturated Fat **0g**

Cholesterol **0mg**

Sodium **2mg**

Carbohydrate **2g**

Dietary Fibre **1g**

Sugar **1g**

Protein **0g**

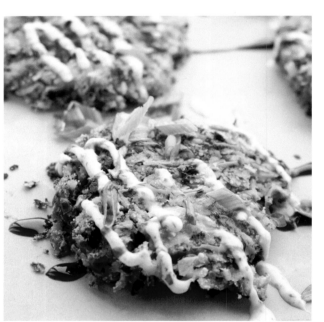
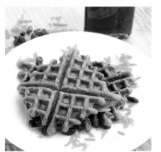
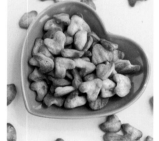

CHAPTER 2

Breakfast

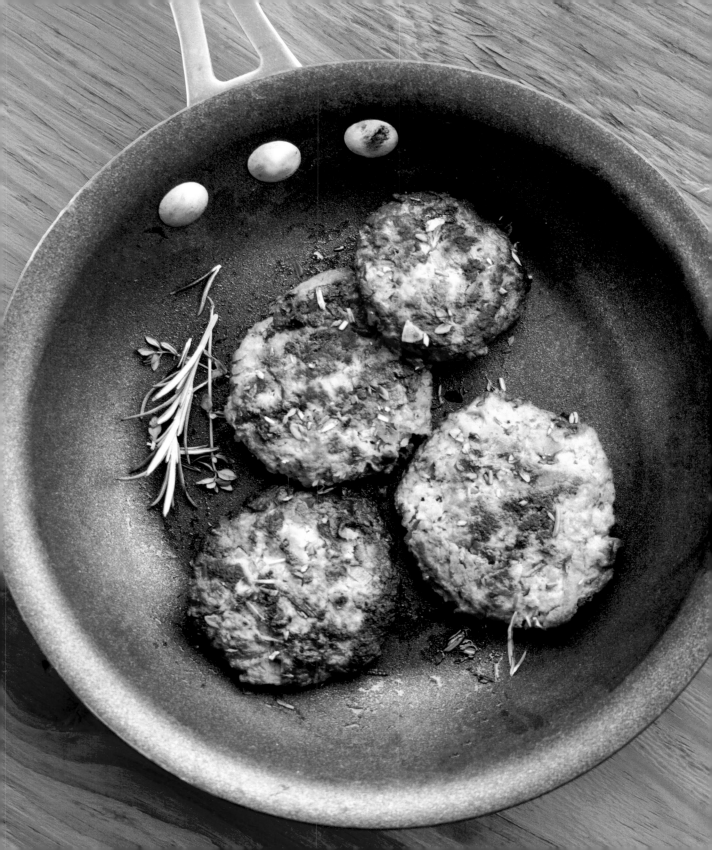

Shredded apples and a **hint of maple syrup** give these herbed pork sausage patties a sweet breakfast flavour.

Rosemary and Thyme
Breakfast Sausage Patties

 YIELD: **12 PATTIES**   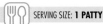 SERVING SIZE: **1 PATTY**   PREP TIME: **10 MINUTES**   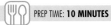 COOK TIME: **10 MINUTES**

INGREDIENTS

- 450g (1 lb.) ground pork
- 1 tbsp maple syrup
- 1 tsp sea salt
- 1 tsp fresh rosemary, chopped
- 1 tsp fresh thyme, chopped
- 1 tbsp fresh sage, chopped
- 240g (8½ oz) Granny Smith apple, peeled and grated (1 large apple)
- 150g (5½ oz) onion, chopped
- 1 clove garlic, finely chopped
- 1 tbsp olive oil

METHOD

1 In a large mixing bowl, combine pork, maple syrup, sea salt, rosemary, thyme, sage, apple, onion, and garlic. With clean hands, mix ingredients until well combined.

2 Shape golf-ball-sized portions of meat mixture into firm patties.

3 Place a fying pan over a medium-high heat. Add olive oil to pan and swirl to coat.

4 Add patties to frying pan in batches, being careful not to crowd the pan. Cover and fry each batch for 3 minutes. Flip and cook on other side for another 3 minutes.

Storage: Sausage patties can be refrigerated for up to 1 week or frozen for up to 3 months.

Serving Suggestion: Serve sausage patties with Root Vegetable Breakfast Hash.

NUTRITION

| Calories **114** | Saturated Fat **3g** | Cholesterol **27mg** | Carbohydrate **4g** | Sugar **3g** |
| Total Fat **8g** | Unsaturated Fat **5g** | Sodium **218mg** | Dietary Fibre **1g** | Protein **6g** |

This **sweet breakfast** staple features cauliflower in place of oats. With flavours of apple, cinnamon, and coconut, it is **perfect for any chilly morning**.

Apple Cinnamon
No-Oat Oatmeal

 YIELD: **80G**   SERVING SIZE: **40G**   PREP TIME: **5 MINUTES**   COOK TIME: **25 MINUTES**

INGREDIENTS

- 325g (11½ oz) cauliflower florets
- 225ml (8fl oz) light coconut milk
- 125ml (4fl oz) unsweetened apple sauce
- 15g (½oz) unsweetened shredded coconut
- 2 tbsp maple syrup
- ½ tsp vanilla extract
- ½ tsp cinnamon
- ⅛ tsp ground cloves
- Dash salt

SPECIAL TOOLS

 FOOD PROCESSOR

METHOD

1 Put cauliflower in a food processor. Pulse until it is finely chopped and has a rice-like consistency.

2 Transfer cauliflower rice to a small saucepan. Add coconut milk, apple sauce, shredded coconut, maple syrup, vanilla extract, cinnamon, cloves, and salt. Stir to combine.

3 Bring contents to the boil over a medium-high heat. Reduce heat to medium-low, cover, and simmer for 20 minutes or until mixture has thickened.

4 Return cauliflower mixture to a clean food processor and process for 30 seconds to create a smoother consistency.

5 Allow porridge to cool for 5 minutes before serving.

Storage: Store in an airtight container and refrigerate for up to 1 week.

Serving Suggestion: Served at room temperature with chopped fresh apples or raisins.

> Save time by cooking in batches. Process the entire head of cauliflower and save 150g (5½oz) servings of cauliflower rice in the refrigerator to create this tasty breakfast with ease throughout the week.

NUTRITION

Calories 202	Saturated Fat 3g	Cholesterol 0mg	Carbohydrate 30g	Sugar 24g
Total Fat 9g	Unsaturated Fat 0g	Sodium 88mg	Dietary Fibre 4g	Protein 1g

Sweet, tart, and silky-smooth, this dairy-free "yogurt" marries nutrient-rich avocados with the delicious flavours of **key lime pie**.

Key Lime Avocado **No'gurt**

 YIELD: **450G**    SERVING SIZE: **150G**   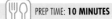 PREP TIME: **10 MINUTES**   COOK TIME: **1 HOUR**

INGREDIENTS

275g (9½oz) avocado (2 medium avocados)

7 tbsp maple syrup

2 tbsp lime juice

1 tbsp lime zest (1 small lime)

SPECIAL TOOLS

 FOOD PROCESSOR

METHOD

1 Cut avocado in half and discard the pit. Scoop avocado flesh from the skin and put in a food processor fitted with a chopping blade.

2 Add maple syrup, lime juice, and lime zest to the food processor. Process for 30 seconds or until smooth.

3 Transfer to a small bowl and refrigerate for 1 hour before serving.

Storage: Store in an airtight container and refrigerate for up to 3 days.

Serving Suggestion: Top No'gurt with unsweetened coconut flakes or fresh berries.

Variation: For Zesty Lemon Avocado No'gurt, substitute lemon juice for lime juice and add lemon zest instead of lime zest.

In addition to their gorgeous green colour, avocados are extremely nutrient-dense, meaning they pack plenty of vitamins, minerals, and phytonutrients into each and every calorie.

NUTRITION

Calories **286**	Saturated Fat **2g**	Cholesterol **0mg**	Carbohydrate **42g**	Sugar **33g**
Total Fat **15g**	Unsaturated Fat **12g**	Sodium **10mg**	Dietary Fibre **7g**	Protein **2g**

This **sweet and crunchy cereal** is made with all AIP-friendly ingredients, including coconut flour, unsweetened **apple sauce**, and ground **cinnamon**.

Apple Cinnamon Hearts **Cereal**

 YIELD: **400G**   SERVING SIZE: **50G**   PREP TIME: **20 MINUTES**   COOK TIME: **15 MINUTES**

INGREDIENTS

55g (2oz) coconut flour

65g (2¼oz) arrowroot powder

50ml (2fl oz) coconut oil

250g (9oz) unsweetened apple sauce

2 tsp vanilla extract

50ml (2fl oz) maple syrup

1 tsp ground cinnamon

SPECIAL TOOLS

 BLENDER

METHOD

1 Preheat oven to 190°C (375°F/Gas 5). Line a baking tray with baking parchment.

2 In a blender, combine coconut flour, arrowroot powder, coconut oil, apple sauce, vanilla, 2 tablespoons maple syrup, and cinnamon. Blend for 30 seconds or until smooth.

3 Transfer batter into a zip-lock bag. Cut a small hole in the corner of the bag to allow the batter to be piped out.

4 Pipe the batter into small heart shapes directly onto the baking parchment, continuing until all batter is used.

5 Bake for 10 minutes. Remove baking tray from the oven and drizzle with additional 2 tablespoons maple syrup. Return to oven and bake for another 5 minutes.

6 Remove baking tray from oven and let cereal cool completely on the tray.

Storage: Store at room temperature in an airtight container for up to 1 week.

Serving Suggestion: Serve with cold coconut milk or as a crunchy topping for Key Lime Avocado No'gurt.

NUTRITION

Calories 159	Saturated Fat 13g	Cholesterol 0mg	Carbohydrate 19g	Sugar 9g
Total Fat 8g	Unsaturated Fat 1g	Sodium 9mg	Dietary Fibre 3g	Protein 2g

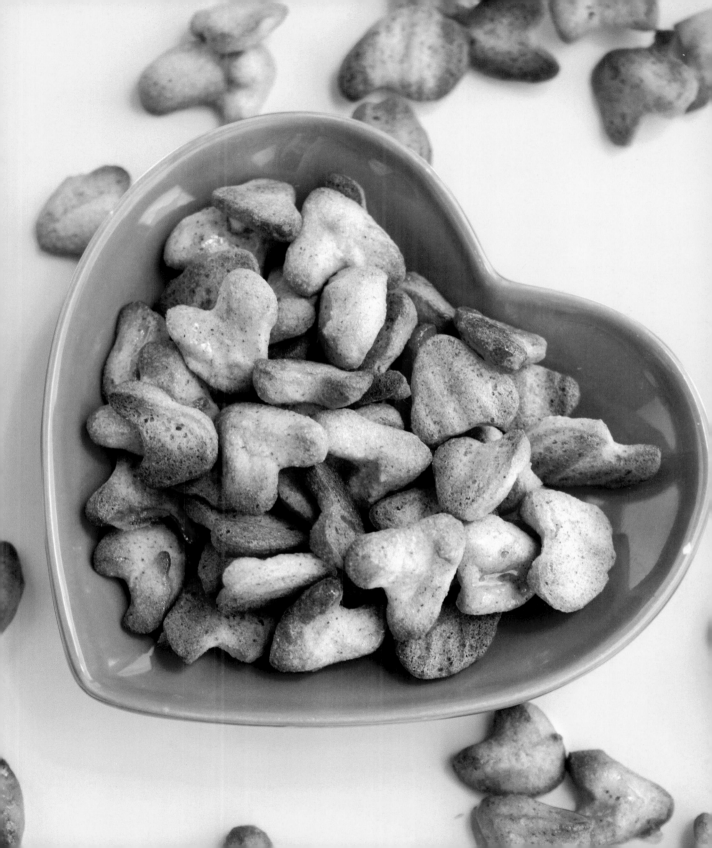

Slices of deli ham are formed into **crisp, savoury cups** perfect for filling with vegetable hash for an easy **grab-and-go breakfast**.

Crisp **Ham Cups**

| YIELD: **12 HAM CUPS** | SERVING SIZE: **2 HAM CUPS** | PREP TIME: **2 MINUTES** | COOK TIME: **20 MINUTES** |

INGREDIENTS

12 slices deli ham

Olive oil nonstick cooking spray

SPECIAL TOOLS

 12-CUP MUFFIN PAN

METHOD

1 Preheat oven to 180°C (350°F/Gas 4).

2 Spray muffin pan with olive oil nonstick cooking spray.

3 Line each muffin cup with a slice of ham, forming the ham into a cup shape.

4 Bake for 10 minutes. Rotate pan and bake for another 10 minutes until crisp and golden brown.

Storage: These are best served crisp right out of the oven, but can be refrigerated for up to 48 hours.

Serving Suggestion: Serve filled with Root Vegetable Breakfast Hash.

NUTRITION

| Calories 82 | Saturated Fat 1g | Cholesterol 35mg | Carbohydrate 35g | Sugar 0g |
| Total Fat 1g | Unsaturated Fat 0g | Sodium 467mg | Dietary Fibre 0g | Protein 14g |

Colourful sweet potatoes, **sweet** carrots, **spicy** parsnips, and **savoury** swede make a nutrient-rich alternative to traditional **hash browns**.

Root Vegetable **Breakfast Hash**

YIELD: **300G**	SERVING SIZE: **75G**	PREP TIME: **10 MINUTES**	COOK TIME: **15 MINUTES**

INGREDIENTS

2 tbsp bacon fat

150g (5½ oz) sweet potato, peeled and chopped

1 tbsp shallot, chopped

150g (5½ oz) onion, chopped (½ onion)

75g (2¾ oz) carrots, peeled and chopped

75g (2¾ oz) parsnips, peeled and chopped

150g (5½ oz) swede, peeled and chopped

1 tsp fresh rosemary, chopped

1 tsp fresh thyme, chopped

½ tsp fresh chives, chopped

⅛ tsp sea salt

METHOD

1 In a large frying pan, heat bacon fat over medium-high heat.

2 Add sweet potato, shallot, onion, carrots, parsnips, and swede.

3 Cook for 10 minutes. Cover pan and continue cooking for another 5 minutes or until vegetables are fork tender.

4 Sprinkle rosemary, thyme, chives, and sea salt over vegetables and stir to combine.

Storage: Refrigerate for up to 3 days or freeze for up to 3 months.

Serving Suggestion: Spoon hash into Crisp Ham Cups for a quick and easy breakfast.

Regular sweet potato can be substituted in this recipe with purple sweet potato, which has deep purple skin and vibrant purple flesh. Use it to brighten up your breakfast instantly!

NUTRITION

Calories **162**	Saturated Fat **3g**	Cholesterol **6mg**	Carbohydrate **24g**	Sugar **5g**
Total Fat **7g**	Unsaturated Fat **4g**	Sodium **103mg**	Dietary Fibre **4g**	Protein **2g**

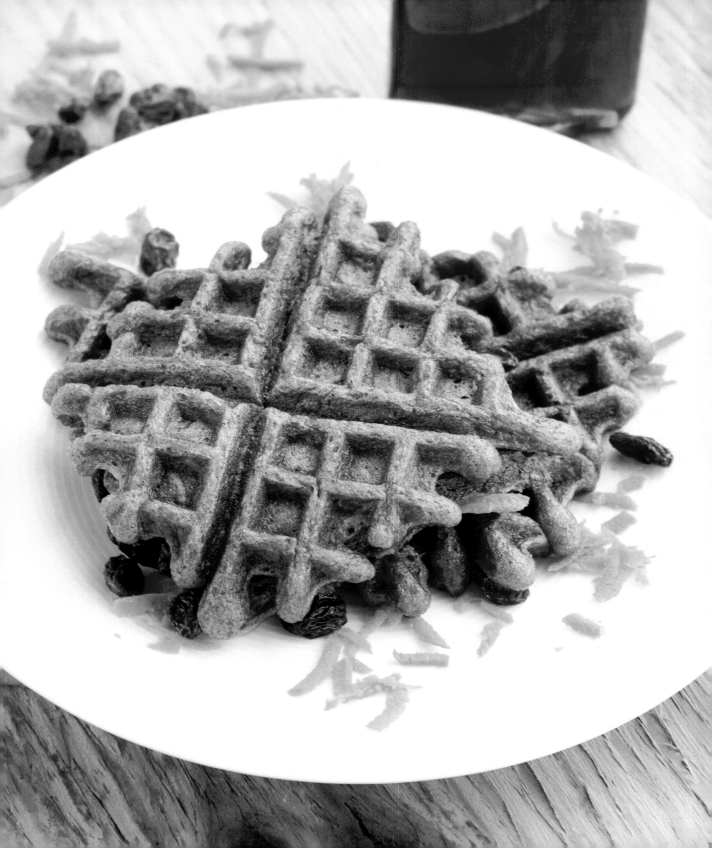

Shredded carrots and raisins bring classic carrot cake flavour to these tender waffles made with plantains, pumpkin purée, and sweet maple syrup.

Carrot Cake **Waffles**

 YIELD: **12 WAFFLES**   SERVING SIZE: **2 WAFFLES**   PREP TIME: **15 MINUTES**   COOK TIME: **2 MINUTES**

INGREDIENTS

- 600g (1lb 5oz) plantains or bananas, peeled and chopped (ripe or green)
- 115g (4oz) pumpkin purée
- 50ml (2fl oz) coconut oil, melted
- 50ml (2fl oz) maple syrup
- 125ml (4fl oz) light coconut milk
- 1 tsp cider vinegar
- 65g (2½oz) arrowroot powder
- 2 tsp bicarbonate of soda
- 1 tsp cream of tartar
- 1 tsp ground cinnamon
- ½ tsp ground ginger
- 1 cup shredded carrots
- ½ cup raisins

SPECIAL TOOLS

 BLENDER

 WAFFLE IRON

METHOD

1 Combine plantains, pumpkin purée, coconut oil, maple syrup, coconut milk, and cider vinegar in a blender. Blend until smooth.

2 Add arrowroot powder, soda, cream of tartar, cinnamon, and ginger to blender. Blend until smooth.

3 Transfer batter to a large bowl. Fold in shredded carrots and raisins.

4 Heat waffle iron to a medium heat. Ladle a portion of batter into the well-greased waffle iron and cook for 2 to 3 minutes. Continue with remaining batter, greasing waffle iron between batches.

Storage: Waffles are best served immediately, but can be stored in the freezer for up to 1 month and reheated in a toaster.

Serving Suggestion: Top waffles with Coconut Whipped Cream or maple syrup.

NUTRITION

Calories **319**	Saturated Fat **16g**	Cholesterol **0mg**	Carbohydrate **56g**	Sugar **30g**
Total Fat **11g**	Unsaturated Fat **1g**	Sodium **445mg**	Dietary Fibre **4g**	Protein **2g**

With **toasted coconut** as a base, this **AIP-friendly breakfast cereal** is free of grains and nuts but retains the texture and flavour of traditional granola.

Sweet and Spicy **Gra'no'la**

 YIELD: **300G**   SERVING SIZE: **50G**   PREP TIME: **5 MINUTES**   COOK TIME: **10 MINUTES**

INGREDIENTS

1 tbsp coconut oil

1 tbsp coconut butter

150g (5½oz) unsweetened coconut flakes

½ tsp cinnamon

¼ tsp sea salt

½ tsp coconut sugar

55g (2oz) unsweetened banana chips, chopped

55g (2oz) unsweetened dried mango, chopped

METHOD

1 Preheat oven to 180°C (350°F/Gas 4).

2 In a small saucepan over a low heat, combine coconut oil and coconut butter. Stir until melted. Remove from heat and set aside.

3 In a large bowl, combine coconut flakes, coconut oil mixture, cinnamon, salt, and coconut sugar. Toss to combine until the flakes are well coated.

4 Line a baking tray with baking parchment. Spread coconut flakes on baking tray and bake for 5 minutes. With a spatula, stir coconut flakes and bake for another 2 to 3 minutes or until golden brown.

5 Remove coconut flakes from oven and transfer to an airtight container. Cool, uncovered, in the fridge or freezer for 10 minutes until dry.

6 Add banana chips and dried mango to coconut flakes. Mix to combine.

Storage: Refrigerate or freeze in a covered, airtight container for up to 1 week.

Serving Suggestion: Sprinkle granola over Key Lime Avocado No'gurt or serve with chilled coconut milk.

NUTRITION

Calories 210	Saturated Fat 10g	Cholesterol 0mg	Carbohydrate 15g	Sugar 10g
Total Fat 13g	Unsaturated Fat 0g	Sodium 116mg	Dietary Fibre 3g	Protein 1g

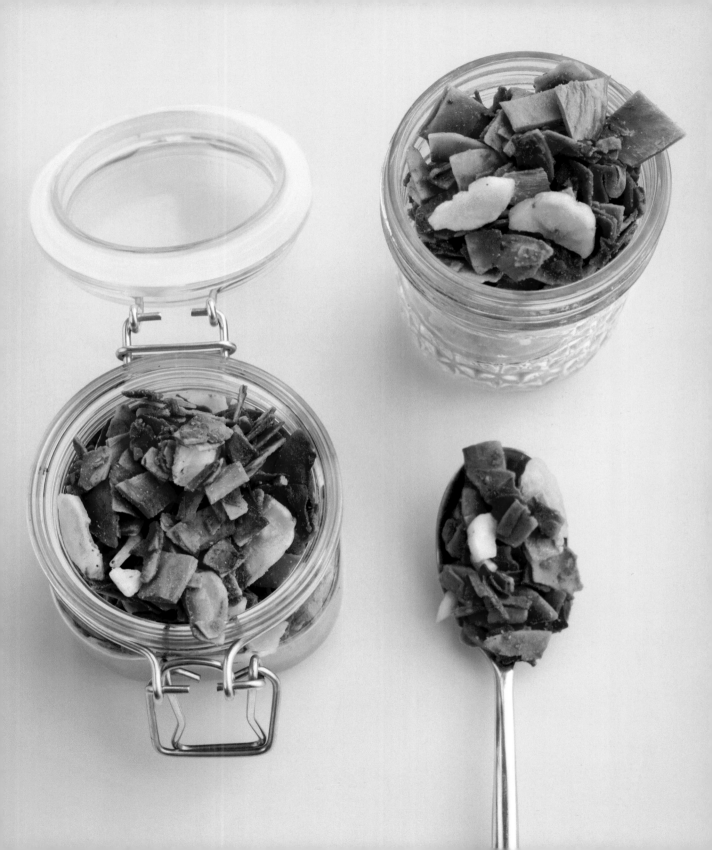

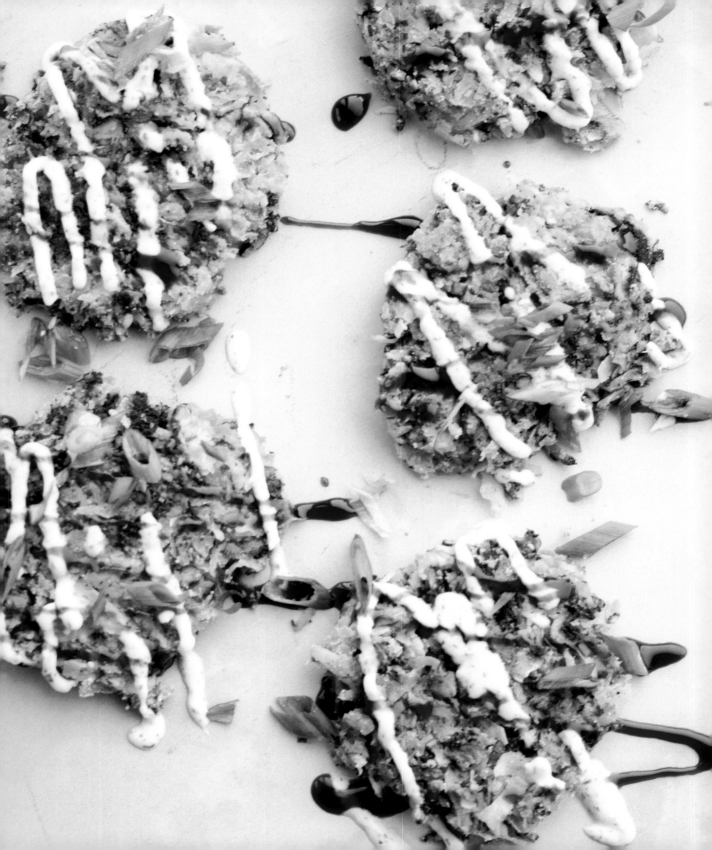

These savoury Japanese **vegetable pancakes** rely on the binding properties of **coconut flour and apple sauce** to form tasty, nutrient-dense fritters.

Okonomiyaki
(Savoury Japanese Pancake)

 YIELD: **10 PANCAKES**   SERVING SIZE: **2 PANCAKES**   PREP TIME: **10 MINUTES**   COOK TIME: **20 MINUTES**

INGREDIENTS

300g (10½oz) cabbage (any variety), shredded

175g (6oz) courgette, shredded

50g (2oz) carrots, shredded

115g (4oz) spring onions, chopped

40g (1½oz) coconut flour

1 tsp arrowroot powder

400ml (14fl oz) light coconut milk

¼ tsp **Seed-Free Curry Powder**

¼ tsp sea salt

¼ tsp garlic powder

85g (3oz) unsweetened apple sauce

1 tbsp coconut oil

METHOD

1 In a large bowl, combine cabbage, courgette, carrots, and spring onions.

2 In a small bowl, combine coconut flour, arrowroot powder, coconut milk, Seed-Free Curry Powder, salt, garlic powder, and apple sauce.

3 Pour the wet ingredients over the vegetable mixture and gently mix to combine.

4 Heat coconut oil in a large frying pan over a medium-high heat. Scoop large spoonfuls of batter into the hot pan.

5 Cook for 5 minutes. Carefully holding the pancakes together, flip and cook for another 5 minutes on the other side until golden brown.

Storage: Okonomiyaki is best served immediately.

Serving Suggestion: Top with Coconut Cream Ranch Dressing and garnish with additional spring onions.

NUTRITION

| Calories 172 | Saturated Fat 8g | Cholesterol 0mg | Carbohydrate 19g | Sugar 8g |
| Total Fat 8g | Unsaturated Fat 0g | Sodium 175mg | Dietary Fibre 7g | Protein 4g |

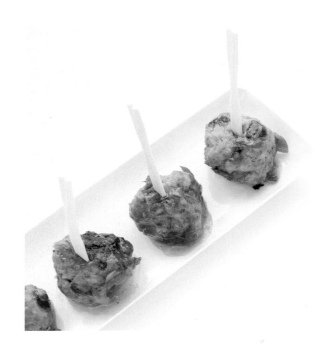
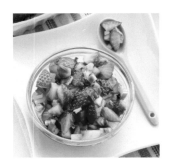
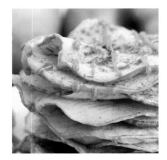

CHAPTER 3
Appetizers
& Snacks

Tangy and sweet apricot preserves pair with the **savoury flavours of ginger and garlic** to create a hearty appetizer perfect for any cocktail party.

Sweet & Sour
Cocktail Meatballs

 YIELD: **32 MEATBALLS**   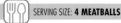 SERVING SIZE: **4 MEATBALLS**   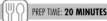 PREP TIME: **20 MINUTES**   COOK TIME: **30 MINUTES**

INGREDIENTS

- 80g (3oz) all-natural apricot preserves
- 4½ tsp Worcestershire Sauce
- ¼ tsp ground ginger
- 3 tbsp coconut aminos
- 1 tbsp olive oil
- 300g (10½oz) green cabbage, thinly chopped
- 50ml (2 fl oz) light coconut milk
- 1½ tsp tapioca starch
- 450g (1 lb) minced pork
- 225g (½ lb) minced veal
- 3 garlic cloves, minced
- 1 tsp fresh ginger, minced
- 60g (2¼oz) spring onion, chopped
- 1 tbsp coconut oil
- Dash sea salt

METHOD

1 In a small saucepan over a medium-high heat, combine apricot preserves, Worcestershire Sauce, ground ginger, and 1 tablespoon coconut aminos. Bring sauce to the boil. Remove from heat, cover, and set aside.

2 Preheat oven to 200°C (400°F/ Gas 6).

3 Heat a large frying pan over a medium-high heat. Add olive oil and cabbage. Sauté for 5 minutes or until cabbage is soft and beginning to brown. Remove from heat.

4 In a large bowl, whisk together coconut milk and tapioca starch.

5 Add cooked cabbage, remaining 2 tablespoons coconut aminos, pork, veal, garlic, ginger, and green onions. With clean hands, mix until well combined.

6 Heat 1 tablespoon coconut oil in a large frying pan over high heat. Scoop 1 tablespoon meat mixture and form into a meatball. Place in hot oil and brown on all sides (about 5 minutes). Continue with remaining meat mixture, working in batches.

7 Line a baking tray with baking parchment. Place browned meatballs on baking tray and brush with apricot sauce. Bake for 15 minutes or until internal temperature reaches 70°C (160°F). Sprinkle with a dash of sea salt before serving.

Storage: Store meatballs in the fridge for up to 1 week or freeze for up to 1 month.

Serving Suggestion: Insert toothpicks and place on a platter as an appetizer or serve over a bed of Cauliflower Fried Rice for an Asian-inspired dinner.

NUTRITION

Calories **309**	Saturated Fat **7g**	Cholesterol **76mg**	Carbohydrate **16g**	Sugar **9g**
Total Fat **18g**	Unsaturated Fat **8g**	Sodium **294mg**	Dietary Fibre **2g**	Protein **21g**

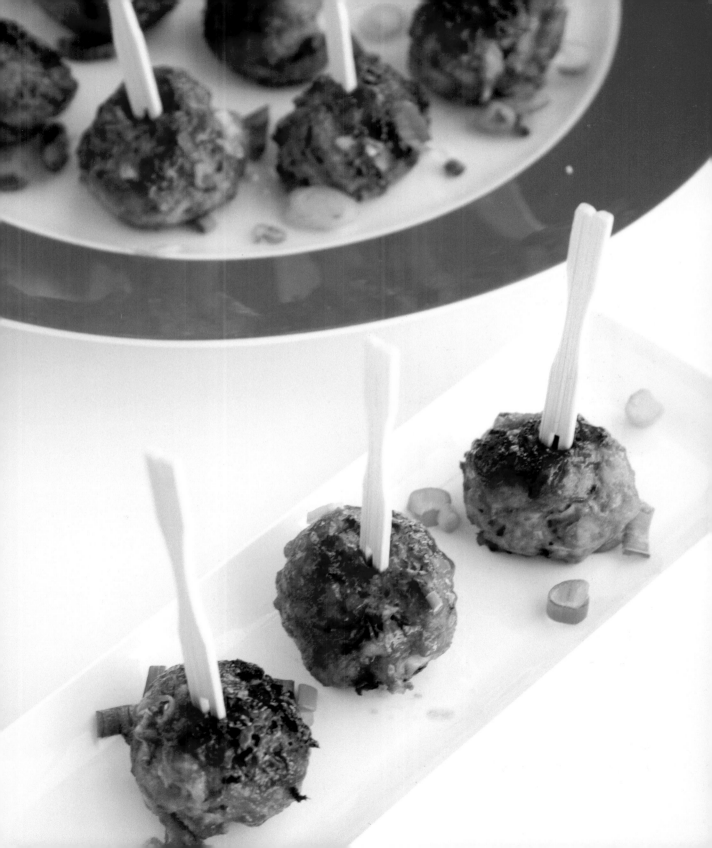

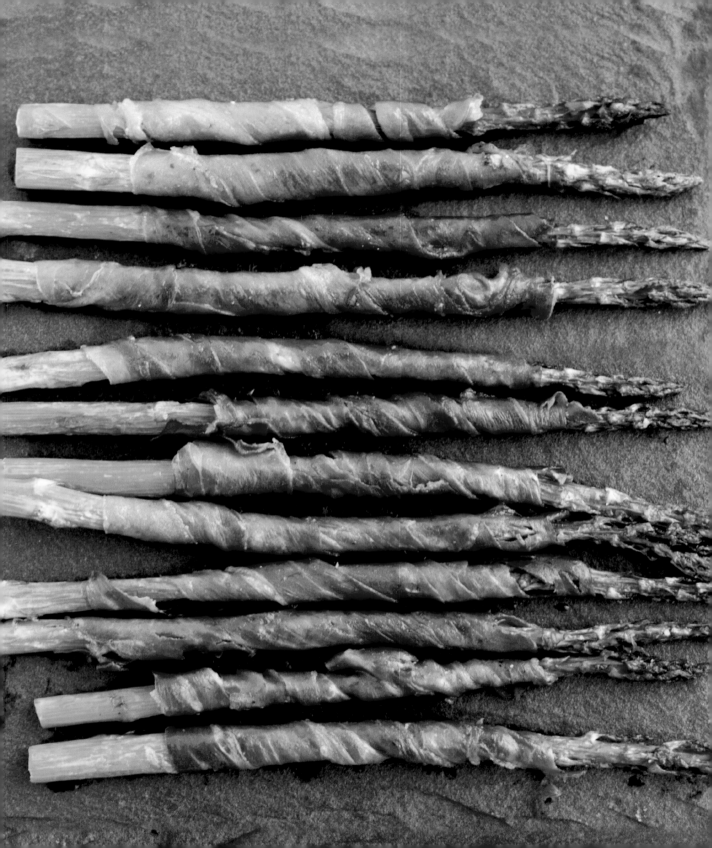

Grilling this easy and elegant finger food creates a **crispy prosciutto** outer layer with a **perfectly tender asparagus** spear inside.

Prosciutto-Wrapped **Asparagus**

 YIELD: **18 SPEARS**   SERVING SIZE: **3 SPEARS**   PREP TIME: **10 MINUTES**   COOK TIME: **10 MINUTES**

INGREDIENTS

- 18 spears asparagus
- 1 tbsp olive oil
- 9 pieces prosciutto, cut lengthwise (about 75g/3 oz)

METHOD

1 Heat the grill to high.

2 Trim the woody ends of the asparagus, leaving the heads intact.

3 In a large bowl, toss asparagus spears with olive oil.

4 Wrap each spear with prosciutto, beginning at the head and rolling the prosciutto at a diagonal to allow for minimal overlap of the prosciutto layers.

5 Line a baking tray with foil. Lay the wrapped asparagus spears on the baking tray, allowing room between them so they do not touch.

6 Grill for 5 minutes, and then flip the spears and grill for another 5 minutes.

7 Remove the tray from the heat and allow spears to cool slightly before serving.

Serving Suggestion: Prosciutto-Wrapped Asparagus spears are best served immediately to maintain their crispness. This dish can be assembled ahead of time and grilled right before you plan on serving it.

Instead of using a knife, trim the ends of the asparagus by hand. Simply bend each spear until it snaps. The less flexible, dry end will break off, leaving just the moist, tasty part of the spear that you want to eat.

NUTRITION

Calories 60
Total Fat 4g
Saturated Fat 1g
Unsaturated Fat 2g
Cholesterol 10mg
Sodium 264mg
Carbohydrate 2g
Dietary Fibre 1g
Sugar 1g
Protein 5g

In this refreshing appetizer, **the sweet flavour of fresh prawns is highlighted with a tangy marinade** of lime juice, vinegar, and creamy avocado.

Citrus Prawn **Ceviche**

 YIELD: **1.8KG**   SERVING SIZE: **300G**   PREP TIME: **10 MINUTES**   CHILL TIME: **I HOUR**

INGREDIENTS

- 1 litre water
- ¼ tsp sea salt
- 4 limes, halved
- 450g (1lb) prawns, peeled and deveined
- 120g (4oz) jicama or Granny Smith apple, peeled and chopped
- 100g (3½oz) spring onions, finely chopped
- 1 tsp dried oregano
- 2 tsp fresh thyme, chopped
- 175ml (6fl oz) lime juice
- 50ml (2fl oz) cider vinegar
- 1 avocado, chopped
- 15g (½oz) fresh coriander, chopped
- ¼ tsp salt

METHOD

1 In a large saucepan over a high heat, combine water and salt. Squeeze juice from lime halves into the water and toss in the lime rinds. Bring contents to a boil.

2 Add prawns and bring contents back to a boil. Remove pan from heat and strain, discarding water and lime rinds.

3 Return hot saucepan to the hob and turn off the heat. Place warm prawns back into the pan, cover, and allow to steam for 5 minutes.

4 Spread prawns on a baking sheet to cool. Remove tails and chop prawns into small pieces.

5 In a large bowl, add prawns, jicama, spring onions, oregano, thyme, lime juice, and cider vinegar. Refrigerate for 1 hour.

6 Add avocado, fresh coriander, and salt to taste before serving.

Storage: Ceviche is best served immediately, but can be refrigerated for up to 3 days.

Serving Suggestion: Serve ceviche on top of sliced cucumbers or with crunchy plantain chips.

NUTRITION

Calories **73**
Total Fat **2g**
Saturated Fat **0g**
Unsaturated Fat **0g**
Cholesterol **0mg**
Sodium **81mg**
Carbohydrate **7g**
Dietary Fibre **2g**
Sugar **2g**
Protein **8g**

This **homemade savoury snack** has the **sweet and salty** flavours you crave without the rapeseed, safflower, or sunflower oil found in most bought crisps.

Rosemary **Sweet Potato Crisps**

 YIELD: **72G**   SERVING SIZE: **18G**   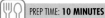 PREP TIME: **10 MINUTES**   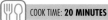 COOK TIME: **20 MINUTES**

INGREDIENTS

- 2 medium sweet potatoes, peeled
- 3 tbsp olive oil
- 2 tbsp fresh rosemary, finely chopped
- ¼ tsp garlic powder
- ⅛ tsp sea salt

SPECIAL TOOLS

 MANDOLIN

METHOD

1 Preheat oven to 190°C (375°F/Gas 5). Line a baking sheet with aluminium foil.

2 Using a mandolin or sharp knife, thinly slice sweet potatoes horizontally into 6mm (¼-inch)-thick slices.

3 In a large bowl, combine sweet potatoes, olive oil, and rosemary. Toss to coat.

4 Place sweet potato slices on baking sheet and sprinkle with garlic powder and sea salt.

5 Bake for 15 minutes. Reduce heat to 180°C (350°F/Gas 4) and bake for another 5 minutes.

Storage: Store sweet potato crisps in an airtight bag or container at room temperature for up to 4 days.

Serving Suggestion: Munch on these chips for a quick snack or dip them in Garlic Herb Avocado Mayo for an easy appetizer.

Variation: Make Thyme Swede Crisps by substituting 2 medium swedes for the sweet potatoes and 2 tablespoons fresh thyme for the rosemary.

A mandolin will create uniformly sized crisps, the key to even cooking. Check on the crisps every few minutes and remove the ones that cook more quickly, leaving the remaining crisps to continue baking.

NUTRITION

Calories **147**
Total Fat **10g**
Saturated Fat **1g**
Unsaturated Fat **8g**
Cholesterol **0mg**
Sodium **109mg**
Carbohydrate **13g**
Dietary Fibre **2g**
Sugar **3g**
Protein **1g**

These **crispy chips** are naturally sweet due to the low and slow baking method. The addition of cinnamon creates the perfect combination of **sugar and spice**.

Cinnamon **Apple Crisps**

 YIELD: **ABOUT 30 CRISPS**   SERVING SIZE: **10 CRISPS**   PREP TIME: **10 MINUTES**   COOK TIME: **3–4 HOURS**

INGREDIENTS

3 large Granny Smith or similar apples

1 tbsp cinnamon

SPECIAL TOOLS

 MANDOLIN

METHOD

1 Preheat oven to 80°C (170°F/Gas ¼). Line a baking tray with baking parchment.

2 Using a mandolin or sharp knife, thinly cut apples horizontally into 5mm (¼-inch) slices.

3 Lay apple slices on the baking tray and generously sprinkle with cinnamon.

4 Bake for 3 to 4 hours, until dry and crispy, flipping the apple slices every 30 minutes.

Storage: Store apple crisps in an airtight bag or container at room temperature for up to 1 week.

Serving Suggestion: These sweet and spicy apple crisps make a perfect snack. Drizzle with Sea Salt Caramel Sauce for a light and healthy dessert to satisfy your sweet tooth.

These apple crisps can also be made using a dehydrator. Simply lay the apples on the dehydrator trays, sprinkle generously with cinnamon, and dehydrate at 70°C (160°F) for 6 hours or until crispy.

NUTRITION

Calories **116**	Saturated Fat **0g**	Cholesterol **0mg**	Carbohydrate **31g**	Sugar **22g**
Total Fat **0g**	Unsaturated Fat **0g**	Sodium **3mg**	Dietary Fibre **6g**	Protein **1g**

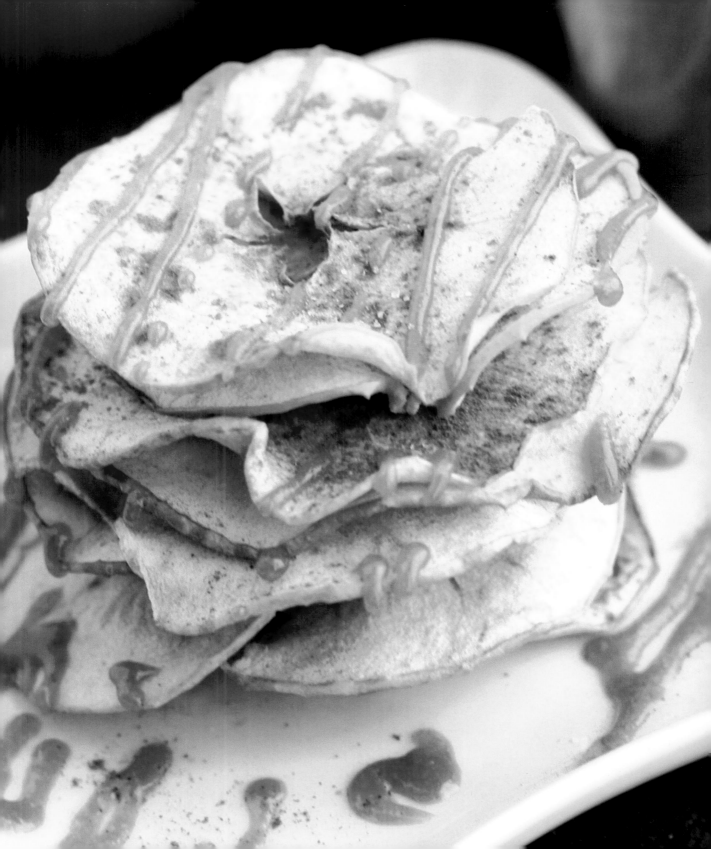

With only **three ingredients**, these nutrient-dense kale crisps are a **crunchy, salty snack food** you can feel good about eating.

Sea Salt **Kale Crisps**

 YIELD: **450G**   SERVING SIZE: **75G**   PREP TIME: **5 MINUTES**   COOK TIME: **10 MINUTES**

INGREDIENTS

1 small bunch kale

3 tbsp olive oil

Dash sea salt

METHOD

1 Preheat oven to 180°C (350°F/Gas 4). Line a baking tray with aluminium foil.

2 Remove kale leaves from stems and tear into 5cm (2-inch) pieces.

3 In a large bowl, combine kale and olive oil. Toss to coat, and then massage the oil into each piece of kale.

4 Spread kale evenly in one layer on baking tray and sprinkle with sea salt.

5 Bake for 10 minutes, flipping the kale chips every 2 minutes.

Storage: Kale crisps are best enjoyed immediately, but can be stored in an airtight container at room temperature for up to 48 hours.

Serving Suggestions: Serve alongside Middle Eastern Bison Burgers and Savoury Baked Butternut Squash at your next barbecue.

NUTRITION

Calories 127	Saturated Fat 1g	Cholesterol 0mg	Carbohydrate 13g	Sugar 0g
Total Fat 8g	Unsaturated Fat 6g	Sodium 84mg	Dietary Fibre 3g	Protein 4g

Balsamic vinegar perfectly complements the **strawberries, cherries, and basil** in this **antioxidant-rich salsa**.

Balsamic Strawberry
Basil Salsa

 YIELD: **900G**   SERVING SIZE: **115G**   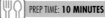 PREP TIME: **10 MINUTES**   COOK TIME: **1 HOUR**

INGREDIENTS

- 600g (1lb 5oz) strawberries, finely chopped
- 225g (½lb) frozen pitted cherries, finely chopped
- 75g (2¾oz) red onion, finely chopped
- 7g (¼oz) fresh basil, chiffonade
- 1 tbsp olive oil
- 1 tbsp balsamic vinegar

METHOD

1 In a large bowl, combine strawberries, cherries, red onion, and basil.

2 Add olive oil and balsamic vinegar and toss to combine.

3 Refrigerate for 1 hour before serving to allow the flavours to meld.

Storage: Store in an airtight container for up to 3 days.

Serving Suggestion: Serve with banana chips or sliced cucumber for an easy appetizer; scoop on grilled salmon or chicken, or add to your favourite salad for a burst of summertime flavour.

Chiffonade is a chopping technique used to cut delicate herbs into long, thin strips. Stack several basil leaves together and roll them up tightly. Slice perpendicular to the roll.

NUTRITION

Calories **41**	Saturated Fat **0g**	Cholesterol **0mg**	Carbohydrate **6g**	Sugar **4g**
Total Fat **2g**	Unsaturated Fat **1g**	Sodium **1mg**	Dietary Fibre **1g**	Protein **1g**

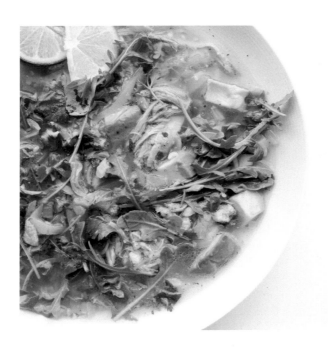
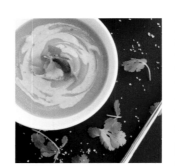
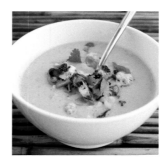

CHAPTER 4
Soups
& Stews

Sweet, caramelized roasted cauliflower is cooked in a rich curry base to create this comforting, Thai-inspired curry cauliflower soup.

Thai **Coconut Curry** Soup

 YIELD: **ABOUT 1 LITRE**   SERVING SIZE: **250ML**   PREP TIME: **30 MINUTES**   COOK TIME: **10 MINUTES**

INGREDIENTS

1 medium head cauliflower, cut into florets

2 tbsp coconut oil

300g (10½oz) onion, chopped (1 large onion)

Juice and zest from 1 lemon

1 tbsp Seed-Free Curry Powder

350ml (12fl oz) vegetable stock

400ml light coconut milk

½ tsp honey

¼ tsp sea salt

1 tbsp fresh coriander, chopped

1 tbsp spring onions, chopped

SPECIAL TOOLS

 BLENDER

METHOD

1 Preheat oven to 200°C (400°F/Gas 6). Line a baking tray with foil.

2 Toss cauliflower florets with 1 tablespoon coconut oil and spread on a baking tray. Bake for 25 minutes or until golden brown.

3 In a large stock pot or Dutch oven, combine 1 tablespoon coconut oil and onion over a medium-high heat. Cook for 3 minutes or until onion begins to soften and become translucent.

4 Add lemon zest, lemon juice, Seed-Free Curry Powder, and 125ml (4fl oz) vegetable stock. Cook for another 2 minutes.

5 Add cauliflower, the remaining vegetable stock, coconut milk, honey, and salt. Stir to combine. Bring mixture to the boil. Remove from heat.

6 Transfer soup to a high-speed blender and blend until smooth.

7 Return soup to pot over low heat and cook until soup begins to thicken (about 2 minutes). Remove from heat and top with fresh coriander and spring onions.

Storage: Store soup in an airtight container in the fridge for 1 week or in freezer for up to 3 months.

Serving Suggestion: Serve soup topped with fresh coriander and spring onions.

NUTRITION

| Calories 189 | Saturated Fat 11g | Cholesterol 0mg | Carbohydrate 16g | Sugar 8g |
| Total Fat 12g | Unsaturated Fat 0g | Sodium 481mg | Dietary Fibre 5g | Protein 4g |

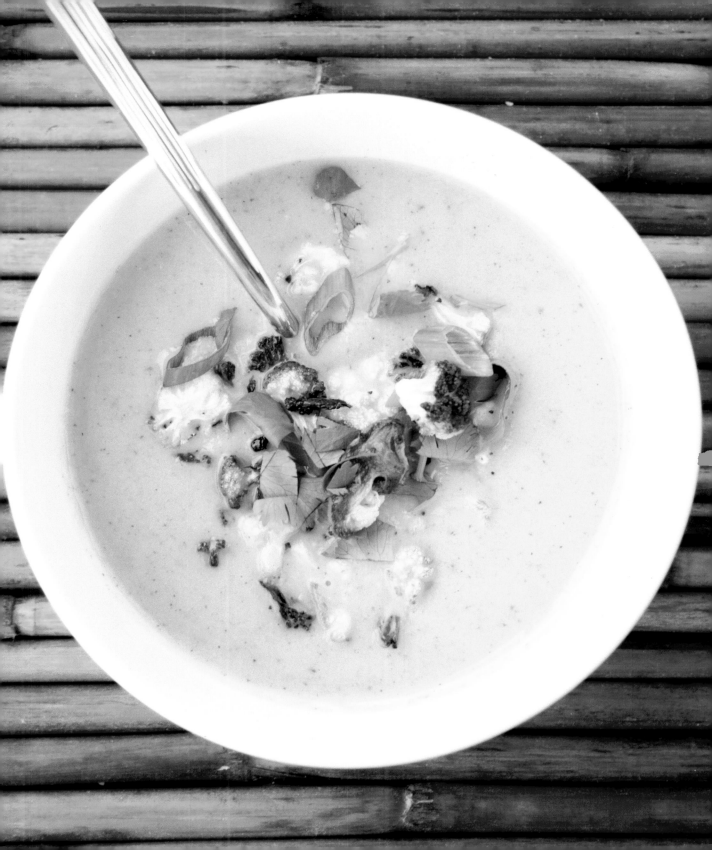

In this **tasty alternative to potato leek soup,** tender roasted cauliflower is puréed into a rich, creamy soup with hints of smoky and tangy flavours.

Cauliflower Leek Soup

 YIELD: **ABOUT 1.3 LITRES**   SERVING SIZE: **325ML**   PREP TIME: **30 MINUTES**   COOK TIME: **20 MINUTES**

INGREDIENTS

1 medium head cauliflower, chopped into florets

1 tbsp coconut oil, melted

1 tbsp bacon fat

180g (6oz) leeks, white and light green parts, sliced (about 2 leeks)

3 slices of bacon, chopped

2 cloves garlic, minced

1 tbsp fresh thyme, chopped

1 tsp white wine vinegar

1 litre (2 pints) chicken stock

50ml (2fl oz) light coconut milk

1 tsp lemon juice

SPECIAL TOOLS

 BLENDER

METHOD

1 Preheat oven to 200°C (400°F/Gas 6). Line a baking tray with foil.

2 Place cauliflower on baking tray and drizzle coconut oil over the cauliflower, massaging it into the florets with clean hands to ensure it is well coated.

3 Bake cauliflower for 15 minutes. Flip the cauliflower and bake for another 10 minutes or until crisp and golden brown. Set aside 80g (3oz) florets for garnish.

4 In a large stock pot or Dutch oven, heat bacon fat over a medium-high heat. Sauté leeks for 10 minutes or until soft and beginning to brown.

5 Add bacon and garlic and cook for another 5 minutes. Add thyme and white wine vinegar and cook for another 2 minutes.

6 Add chicken stock and cooked cauliflower. Bring contents to a boil and then cover and reduce heat. Simmer for 10 minutes. Add coconut milk and lemon juice. Stir to combine.

7 Ladle half of the soup into a high-speed blender. Blend until smooth. Combine blended contents with the remaining soup.

Storage: Store soup in an airtight container in the fridge for 1 week or in the freezer for up to 3 months.

Serving Suggestion: Top soup with roasted cauliflower, chopped chives, or bacon bits.

NUTRITION

Calories **165**

Total Fat **11g**

Saturated Fat **6g**

Unsaturated Fat **3g**

Cholesterol **7mg**

Sodium **865mg**

Carbohydrate **14g**

Dietary Fibre **4g**

Sugar **5g**

Protein **5g**

This soup is **bursting with layers of savoury, authentic flavour.** You won't even miss the traditional bread and cheese.

French Onion Soup

 YIELD: **ABOUT 1 LITRE**   SERVING SIZE: **225ML** 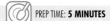 PREP TIME: **5 MINUTES**   COOK TIME: **1 HOUR**

INGREDIENTS

3 onions, thinly sliced

1 tbsp olive oil

¼ tsp sea salt

1 clove garlic, minced

1 tbsp fresh thyme, diced

1 tsp red wine

1 tsp white wine vinegar

1 tsp balsamic vinegar

1 tsp Worcestershire Sauce

1 litre (1¾ pints) beef stock

METHOD

1 In a large stock pot or Dutch oven over a high heat, combine onions, olive oil, and sea salt.

2 Cook for 30 minutes or until onions are dark and caramelized, stirring frequently and adding a splash of beef stock occasionally to prevent onions from burning.

3 Add garlic and thyme. Cook for another 2 minutes.

4 Add red wine, white wine vinegar, and balsamic vinegar. Cook for another 2 minutes until alcohol has burned off.

5 Add Worcestershire Sauce and beef stock. Bring contents to a boil. Reduce heat to low and simmer, partially covered, for 25 minutes.

Storage: Store soup in an airtight container in the fridge for 1 week or in the freezer for up to 3 months.

Serving Suggestion: Stir in some chopped Greek-Style Roast Chicken, Sunday Slow Cooker Pot Roast, or Orange Pulled Pork Carnitas for added protein.

NUTRITION

Calories **159**

Total Fat **3g**

Saturated Fat **0g**

Unsaturated Fat **2g**

Cholesterol **0mg**

Sodium **749mg**

Carbohydrate **8g**

Dietary Fibre **5g**

Sugar **0g**

Protein **3g**

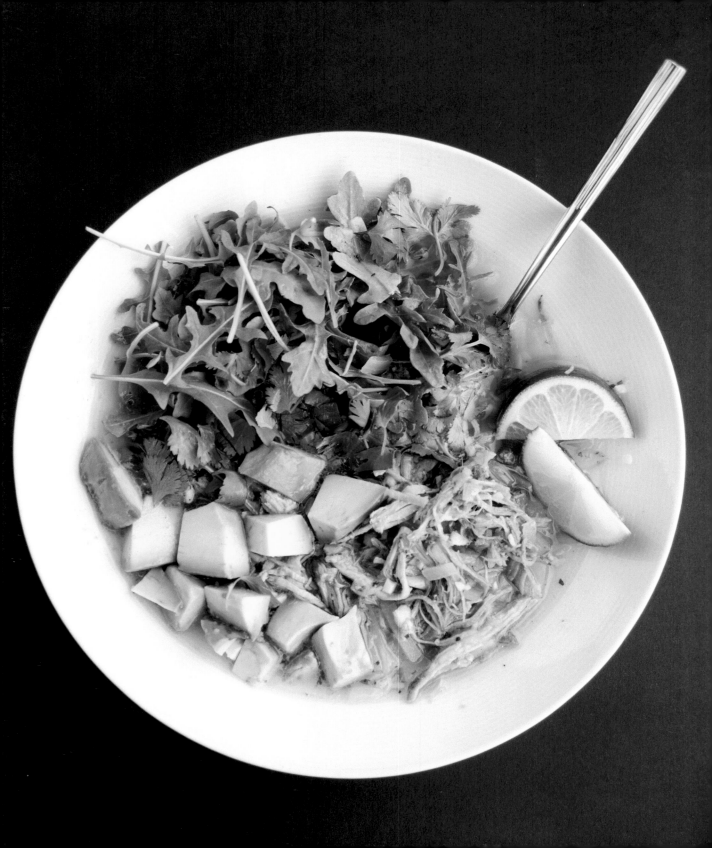

Savour the rich flavours of **slow-cooked shredded pork and garlic** with the freshness of lime, coriander, rocket, and avocado.

Mexican Carnitas
Broth Bowl

 YIELD: **ABOUT 1.4 LITRES**   SERVING SIZE: **225ML**   PREP TIME: **10 MINUTES**   COOK TIME: **40 MINUTES**

INGREDIENTS

2 tbsp olive oil

1 large onion white onion,

1 medium chayote squash (or courgette), peeled, core removed, and chopped

6 garlic cloves, minced

1 litre (about 2 pints) chicken stock

1kg (2lb 4oz) Orange Pulled Pork Carnitas

3 tbsp lime juice

Dash sea salt

2 cups rocket

½ cup fresh coriander

1 avocado, chopped

METHOD

1 In a large stock pot or Dutch oven, heat olive oil, onion, and chayote over a medium-high heat. Sauté for 5 minutes or until vegetables are soft.

2 Add garlic and sauté for another 2 minutes until fragrant.

3 Add chicken broth and Orange Pulled Pork Carnitas. Bring to a boil. Reduce heat, cover, and simmer for 30 minutes.

4 Stir in lime juice and salt. When ready to serve, ladle soup into bowls, top with rocket, fresh coriander, and avocado.

Storage: Store carnitas broth separate from rocket, coriander, and avocado. When ready to enjoy, stir the fresh ingredients into the hot broth. Refrigerate soup for up to 1 week or freeze for up to 3 months.

Originally from Mexico, chayote squash is now enjoyed in many cultures. It has white flesh, a crisp texture, and a mild sweet flavour. Cook it like summer squash, or enjoy it raw in salads or salsas.

NUTRITION

Calories **455**	Saturated Fat **10g**	Cholesterol **94mg**	Carbohydrate **9g**	Sugar **2g**
Total Fat **36g**	Unsaturated Fat **23g**	Sodium **547mg**	Dietary Fibre **4g**	Protein **24g**

Cooking the mushrooms low and slow creates a meaty texture that pairs perfectly with the **deep flavours of beef broth and pork sausage**.

Wild Mushroom
Sausage Stew

 YIELD: **ABOUT 1.4 LITRES**   SERVING SIZE: **225ML**   PREP TIME: **10 MINUTES**   COOK TIME: **1 HOUR**

INGREDIENTS

800g (1lb 12oz) mushrooms, chopped

300g (10½oz) onion, chopped

2 garlic cloves, minced

2 tbsp fresh thyme, chopped

4 tbsp ghee

900ml (1½ pints) beef stock

225g (8oz) pork sausages, thickly sliced

15g (½oz) parsley, chopped

SPECIAL TOOLS

 BLENDER

METHOD

1 In a frying pan, fry the sausage pieces until cooked through. Set aside.

2 In a large saucepan or Dutch oven over a medium-high heat, combine mushrooms, onion, garlic, thyme, and ghee.

3 Cook for 30 minutes, stirring occasionally until mushrooms have released all of their liquid and begin to caramelize.

4 Add beef stock and bring to a boil. Reduce heat, cover, and simmer for 20 minutes.

5 Ladle 225ml (8fl oz) of the soup into blender and blend until smooth. Return puréed soup to pot and combine with remaining soup.

6 Add cooked sausage pieces and bring soup to a boil. Remove from heat and stir in parsley.

Storage: Store soup in an airtight container in the fridge for 1 week or in the freezer for up to 3 months.

NUTRITION

Calories 240	Saturated Fat 9g	Cholesterol 43mg	Carbohydrate 10g	Sugar 4g
Total Fat 19g	Unsaturated Fat 9g	Sodium 439mg	Dietary Fibre 3g	Protein 9g

The **fresh flavours of asparagus and broccoli** are highlighted by smoky bacon and creamy coconut milk in this savoury spring soup.

Spring Asparagus and
Broccoli Bisque

 YIELD: **1 LITRE**   SERVING SIZE: **250ML**   PREP TIME: **20 MINUTES**   COOK TIME: **15 MINUTES**

INGREDIENTS

450g (1lb) asparagus, ends trimmed

500g (1lb 2oz) broccoli florets

1 tbsp olive oil

⅛ tsp sea salt

1 tbsp bacon fat

75g (3oz) shallot, chopped

2 cloves garlic, minced

450ml (16fl oz) vegetable stock

225ml (8fl oz) light coconut milk

2 tbsp lemon juice

SPECIAL TOOLS

 BLENDER

METHOD

1 Preheat oven to 190°C (375°F). Line a baking tray with foil.

2 Place asparagus and broccoli on baking tray. Drizzle with olive oil and massage oil into vegetables until coated. Sprinkle with sea salt. Roast vegetables for 20 minutes.

3 In a large saucepan or Dutch oven, heat bacon fat over medium-high heat. Add shallots and garlic. Cook for 5 minutes or until soft.

4 Add vegetable stock, coconut milk, and lemon juice. Bring contents to the boil. Remove pan from heat.

5 In a blender, combine asparagus, broccoli, and stock. Blend for 30 seconds or until smooth.

6 Return soup to pot and warm over low heat before serving.

Storage: Store soup in an airtight container in the fridge for 1 week or in the freezer for up to 3 months.

NUTRITION

Calories **164**	Saturated Fat **2g**	Cholesterol **3mg**	Carbohydrate **17g**	Sugar **5g**
Total Fat **10g**	Unsaturated Fat **5g**	Sodium **393mg**	Dietary Fibre **6g**	Protein **5g**

This healthy and rustic stew features **hearty bites of sweet butternut squash,** savoury pork sausage, and crunchy kale.

Tuscan **Sausage and Kale** Stew

 YIELD: **ABOUT 1 LITRE**   SERVING SIZE: **225ML**   PREP TIME: **5 MINUTES**   COOK TIME: **40 MINUTES**

INGREDIENTS

1 tbsp olive oil

225g (½ lb) pork sausage, sliced

1 large white onion, chopped

2 cloves garlic, minced

200g (7oz) butternut squash, peeled and chopped

2 bay leaves

1 tsp dried oregano

900ml (1½ pints) chicken stock

50g (2oz) canned sweet potato purée

140g (5oz) kale, stems removed and chopped

METHOD

1 In a large saucepan or Dutch oven, heat olive oil over a medium-high heat. Add sausage, onion, and garlic. Cook for 5 minutes or until meat is no longer pink and vegetables are soft.

2 Add butternut squash and cook for another 10 minutes until vegetables are caramelized and sausage is golden brown.

3 Add bay leaves, oregano, and chicken stock. Bring to a boil.

4 Reduce heat and cover. Simmer stew for 30 minutes.

5 Stir in sweet potato purée and kale. Cook for another 5 minutes or until kale is slightly wilted.

Storage: Store soup in an airtight container in the fridge for 1 week or in the freezer for up to 3 months.

NUTRITION

| Calories 245 | Saturated Fat 4g | Cholesterol 24mg | Carbohydrate 18g | Sugar 3g |
| Total Fat 15g | Unsaturated Fat 9g | Sodium 1,084mg | Dietary Fibre 1g | Protein 9g |

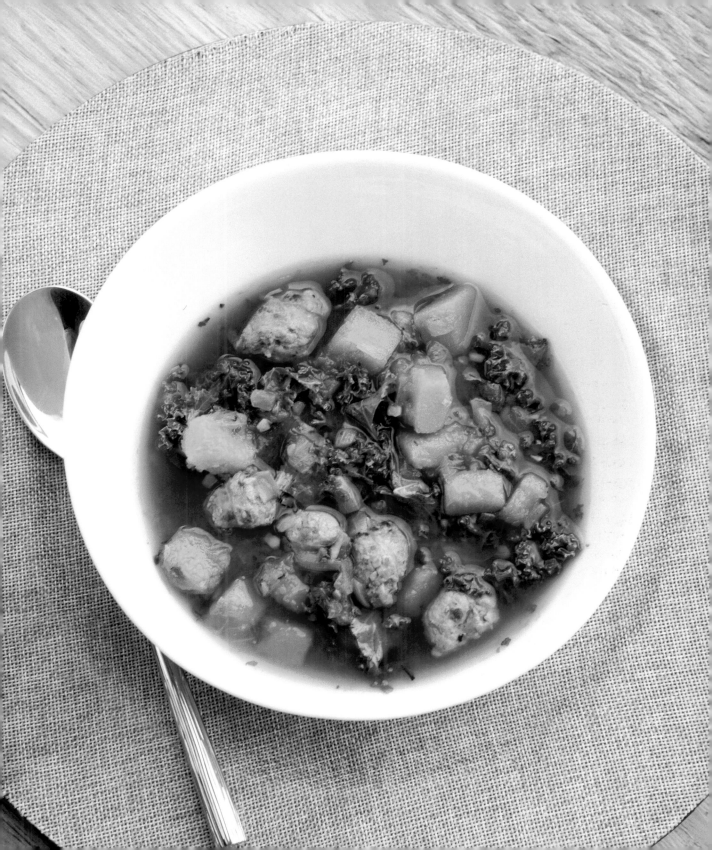

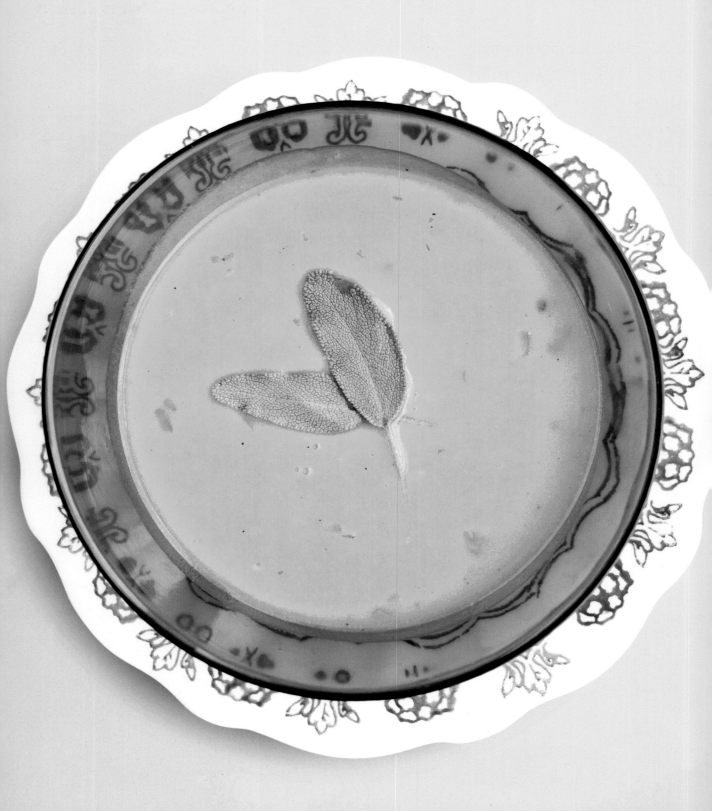

In this **elegant autumn soup,** hearty roasted butternut squash is puréed and paired with a subtle sage cream.

Roasted **Butternut Squash and Sage** Soup

 YIELD: **ABOUT 1.4 LITRES**   SERVING SIZE: **225ML**   PREP TIME: **10 MINUTES**   COOK TIME: **30 MINUTES**

INGREDIENTS

- 1.2kg (2lb 12oz) butternut squash, peeled and cubed
- 2 tbsp olive oil
- ⅛ tsp sea salt
- 225ml (8fl oz) light coconut milk
- 3 tbsp fresh sage, chopped
- 2 tbsp ghee
- 150g (5½oz) shallots, chopped
- 2 garlic cloves, minced
- 900ml (1½ pints) **Bone Broth** (or chicken stock)

SPECIAL TOOLS

 BLENDER

METHOD

1 Preheat oven to 200°C (400°F/Gas 6). Line a baking tray with foil. Spread butternut squash on baking tray, massage with olive oil, and sprinkle with sea salt.

2 Roast squash for 15 minutes. Turn squash, and bake for another 15 minutes. Remove from oven and set aside.

3 In a large saucepan or Dutch oven, heat coconut milk over a medium-high heat. Add sage and stir. Bring to the boil. Transfer contents into a small bowl and set aside for 10 minutes to steep.

4 In a clean saucepan, heat ghee over a medium-high heat. Add shallots and garlic. Cook for 2 to 3 minutes or until soft.

5 Add roasted butternut squash and Bone Broth. Bring contents to a boil. Reduce heat and simmer, covered, for 10 minutes.

6 Transfer contents to a high-speed blender. Blend contents until smooth.

7 Return soup to saucepan and stir in the coconut milk and sage mixture.

Storage: Store soup in an airtight container in the refrigerator for 1 week or in the freezer for up to 3 months.

Variation: To make Spiced Carrot Soup, replace butternut squash with chopped carrots and replace sage with fresh grated ginger.

NUTRITION

Calories **240**
Total Fat **13g**
Saturated Fat **4g**
Unsaturated Fat **6g**
Cholesterol **16mg**
Sodium **88mg**
Carbohydrate **23g**
Dietary Fibre **5g**
Sugar **4g**
Protein **7g**

This hearty puréed soup is **topped with a tangy garlic herb chermoula sauce,** a classic Moroccan sauce traditionally used to top fish and chicken.

Moroccan **Sweet Potato** Soup

 YIELD: **ABOUT 1.4 LITRES**   SERVING SIZE: **225ML**   PREP TIME: **10 MINUTES**   COOK TIME: **30 MINUTES**

INGREDIENTS

- 2 tbsp olive oil
- 1 large onion, chopped
- 1 medium sweet potato, peeled and chopped
- 2–3 medium parsnips, peeled and chopped
- 2–3 medium carrots carrots, peeled and chopped
- 1 tbsp fresh ginger, peeled and minced
- 9 cloves garlic, minced
- 1 tbsp Seed-Free Curry Powder
- 900ml (1½ pints) vegetable stock
- Juice of 2 lemons
- 25g (1 oz) fresh coriander, leaves and stems, chopped
- 15g (½oz) cup parsley
- 50ml (2fl oz) coconut milk

SPECIAL TOOLS

 BLENDER

METHOD

1 Heat olive oil in large saucepan or Dutch oven over a medium-high heat.

2 Add onion, sweet potato, parsnips, carrots, ginger, and 3 teaspoons minced garlic. Sauté for 5 minutes or until onion begins to soften.

3 Add Seed-Free Curry Powder and 125ml (4fl oz) stock. Cook for another 2 minutes until fragrant.

4 Add remaining vegetable stock and bring contents to a boil. Reduce heat to low, cover, and simmer for 30 minutes.

5 Remove from heat and transfer contents to a blender. Blend on high until smooth. Return soup to saucepan.

6 In a clean blender, combine remaining minced garlic, lemon juice, fresh coriander, parsley, and coconut milk to make chermoula sauce. Blend until smooth.

7 Stir 1 tablespoon chermoula sauce into each serving of soup.

Storage: Store soup and chermoula sauce separately in the fridge for up to 1 week or in the freezer up to 3 months.

Serving Suggestion: Serve soup topped with chermoula sauce and additional fresh coriander.

NUTRITION

Calories **155**
Total Fat **7g**
Saturated Fat **2g**
Unsaturated Fat **4g**
Cholesterol **0mg**
Sodium **429mg**
Carbohydrate **22g**
Dietary Fibre **4g**
Sugar **5g**
Protein **2g**

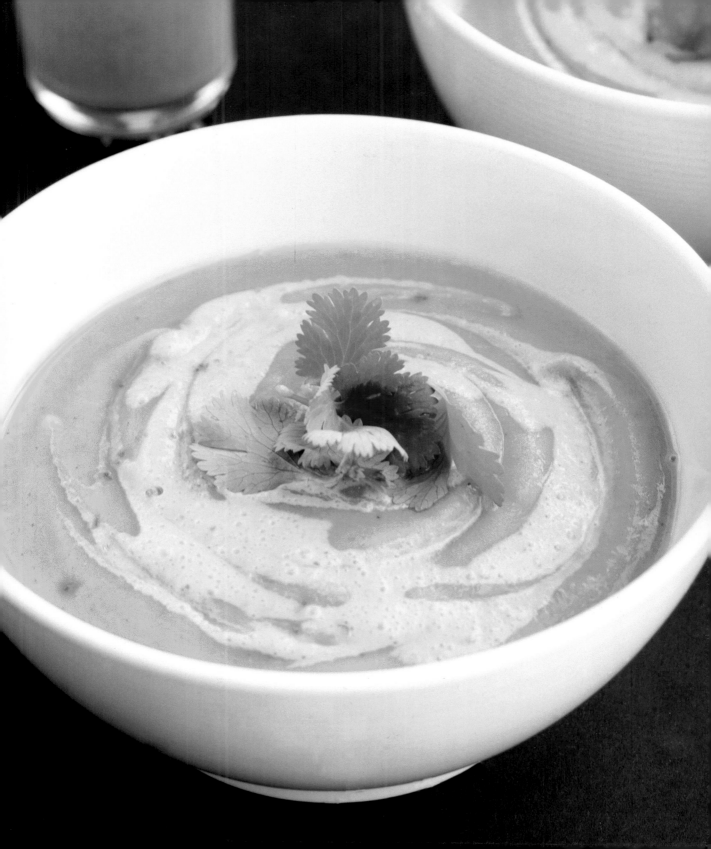

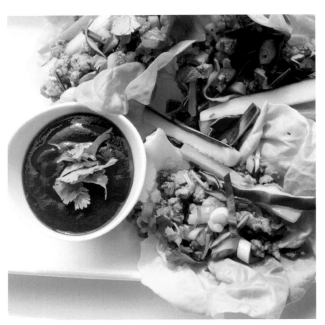

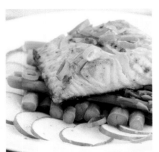

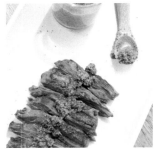

CHAPTER 5
Main Courses

With flavours of ginger and orange zest, a quick and easy marinade gives this **omega-3 rich salmon** a sweet, tangy citrus glaze.

Honey Ginger
Glazed Salmon

 YIELD: **4 FILLETS** 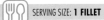 SERVING SIZE: **1 FILLET** PREP TIME: **1 HOUR** COOK TIME: **15 MINUTES**

INGREDIENTS

- 50ml (2fl oz) orange juice
- 50ml (2fl oz) honey
- 50ml (2fl oz) coconut aminos
- 1 tbsp olive oil
- 4 spring onions, sliced
- 1 tbsp fresh ginger, peeled
- 1 tbsp sherry vinegar
- ½ tsp orange zest
- 4 x 112g (4oz) salmon fillets, skin on

SPECIAL TOOLS

 FOOD PROCESSOR

METHOD

1 In a food processor, combine orange juice, honey, coconut aminos, olive oil, spring onions, ginger, sherry vinegar, and orange zest. Process for 30 seconds or until well combined.

2 Pour marinade into a zip-lock plastic bag. Add salmon and seal. Refrigerate and marinate salmon for 1 hour.

3 Heat a medium frying pan over a medium-high heat. Add salmon to hot pan, skin-side down. Spoon 50ml (2fl oz) marinade over the salmon. Allow to cook for 3 minutes.

4 Flip salmon and cook for another 3 minutes or until salmon is flaky and cooked through.

Storage: Salmon is best served immediately, but leftovers can be refrigerated and used for lunch or dinner the following day.

Serving Suggestion: Serve salmon over leafy greens or vegetable of your choice and garnish with sliced spring onions.

NUTRITION

Calories **249**	Saturated Fat **1g**	Cholesterol **59mg**	Carbohydrate **22g**	Sugar **19g**
Total Fat **7g**	Unsaturated Fat **6g**	Sodium **412mg**	Dietary Fibre⁰ **0g**	Protein **23g**

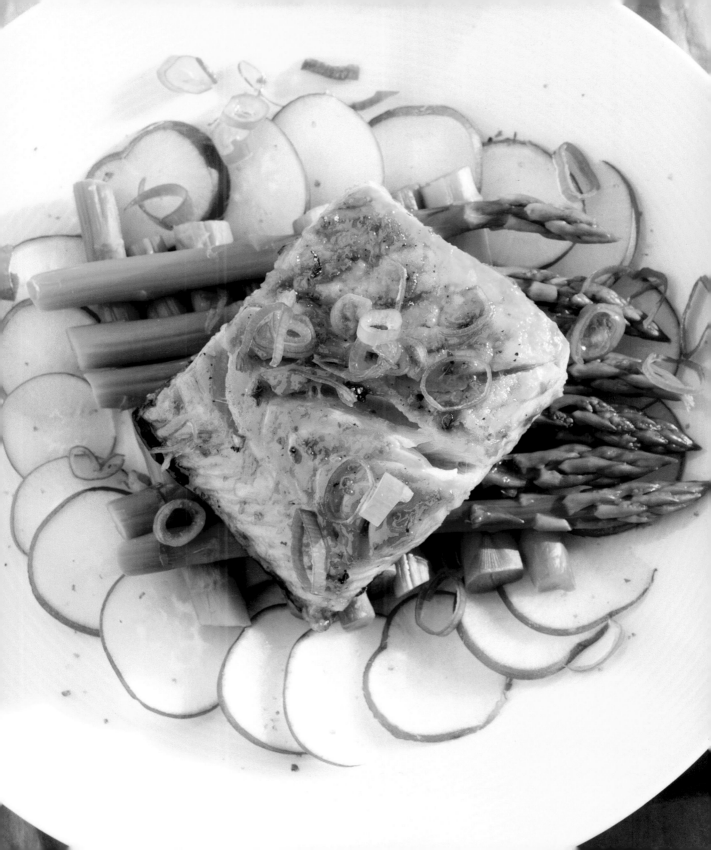

This garlic-infused pot roast becomes deliciously tender in the slow cooker. With a tangy shallot sauce, it's **comfort food at its best**.

Sunday Slow Cooker **Pot Roast**

 YIELD: **8 SLICES** 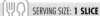 SERVING SIZE: **1 SLICE** PREP TIME: **10 MINUTES** COOK TIME: **7 HOURS**

INGREDIENTS

- 3–4 parsnips, peeled and chopped
- 1 large sweet potato, peeled and chopped
- 300g (10½ oz) shallots, chopped
- 1.5kg (3lb) boneless braising steak
- 8 cloves garlic, thinly sliced
- 1½ tsp sea salt
- 350ml (12fl oz) beef stock
- 2 tbsp Worcestershire Sauce
- 2 tsp lemon juice
- 50ml (2fl oz) ghee, melted
- 1 tbsp tapioca starch
- 15g (½ oz) parsley, chopped

SPECIAL TOOLS

 SLOW COOKER

METHOD

1 Put the parsnips, sweet potatoes, and shallots at the bottom of a slow cooker.

2 Using a paring knife, make small cuts into both sides of the meat. Insert garlic slices into the cuts and season the meat with 1 teaspoon sea salt.

3 Put seasoned braising steak into slow cooker, nestling it among the vegetables.

4 In a small bowl, whisk together beef stock, Worcestershire Sauce, lemon juice, and remaining ½ teaspoon sea salt. Pour sauce into slow cooker over the meat.

5 Cover and cook meat and vegetables in slow cooker on low for 7 hours.

6 Remove the meat and vegetables from the slow cooker with a slotted spoon.

7 In a small bowl, whisk together ghee, tapioca starch, and parsley. Add contents to the juices in the slow cooker and stir to combine.

8 Slice the meat and spoon the slow-cooker sauce over meat and vegetables.

Storage: Refrigerate pot roast for 5 days or freeze for up to 3 months.

Serving Suggestion: Serve sliced pot roast over vegetables and spoon sauce over the top before serving.

NUTRITION

| Calories **369** | Saturated Fat **4g** | Cholesterol **74mg** | Carbohydrate **23g** | Sugar **4g** |
| Total Fat **22g** | Unsaturated Fat **8g** | Sodium **726mg** | Dietary Fibre **3g** | Protein **18g** |

Beef and broccoli are coated with a **sweet-and-salty ginger garlic sauce** in this dish that mimics familiar restaurant-style flavours.

Broccoli Beef Stir-Fry

 YIELD: **600G**   SERVING SIZE: **150G**   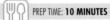 PREP TIME: **10 MINUTES**   COOK TIME: **20 MINUTES**

INGREDIENTS

1 tbsp olive oil

½ large onion, chopped

450g (1lb) skirt steak, thinly sliced

50ml (2fl oz) water

700g (1lb 9oz) broccoli, chopped

125ml (4fl oz) coconut aminos

125ml (4fl oz) beef stock

5 garlic cloves, minced

1 tsp fresh ginger, minced

2 tbsp fish sauce

1 tsp honey

1 tsp tapioca starch

METHOD

1 Heat olive oil in a large frying pan over a medium-high heat. Add onion and cook for 5 minutes or until soft and translucent.

2 Add steak and cook for 5 minutes, flipping occasionally to brown on both sides.

3 Remove steak and onions from frying pan and set aside. Add water and broccoli.

4 Cover and steam for 3 minutes until soft. Remove broccoli from pan.

5 In a small bowl, whisk together coconut aminos, beef stock, garlic, ginger, fish sauce, honey, and tapioca starch.

6 Add sauce to the frying pan and whisk over a medium heat until bubbling and beginning to thicken. Return meat and broccoli to pan and toss to coat.

Storage: Refrigerate for up to 5 days.

Serving Suggestion: Serve over Cauliflower Fried Rice and top with chopped spring onions.

NUTRITION

Calories 313	Saturated Fat 8g	Cholesterol 49mg	Carbohydrate 18g	Sugar 5g
Total Fat 16g	Unsaturated Fat 1g	Sodium 890mg	Dietary Fibre 3g	Protein 24g

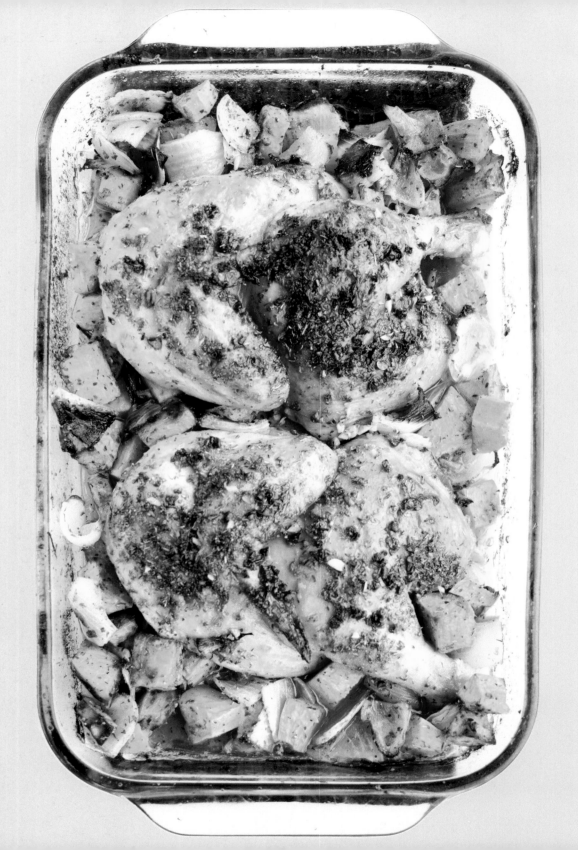

This traditional Greek-style roast chicken is **coated in savoury olive oil and tangy lemon juice** and generously sprinkled with flavourful oregano.

Greek-Style **Roast Chicken**

 YIELD: **8 PIECES**   SERVING SIZE: **1 PIECE**   PREP TIME: **20 MINUTES**   COOK TIME: **1 HOUR 20 MIN**

INGREDIENTS

- 2.1kg (4.5lb) roasting chicken, without giblets
- Juice of 3 lemons
- 125ml (4fl oz) olive oil
- ¼ tsp sea salt
- ¼ tsp garlic powder
- ¼ tsp onion powder
- 2 tbsp dried oregano
- 10 cloves garlic, minced
- 1 large yellow onion, quartered
- 2 medium sweet potatoes, cubed

METHOD

1 Preheat oven to 190°C (375°F/Gas 5). Line the bottom of a baking dish with baking parchment.

2 Rinse chicken under cold water and pat dry with kitchen towels. Using a sharp knife or poultry shears, cut chicken in half along the backbone. Discard the backbone and lay the two chicken halves on the baking parchment.

3 Pour the lemon juice over the chicken halves, rubbing it into the skin.

4 Drizzle 50ml (2fl oz) olive oil over the chicken, massaging it into the chicken.

5 In a small bowl, combine salt, garlic powder, onion powder, and oregano.

6 Season chicken halves with half of the seasoning mixture.

7 In a large bowl, combine garlic, onion, sweet potatoes, remaining olive oil, and remaining half of seasoning mixture. Toss to combine. Spread onion and sweet potatoes mixture around the chicken halves.

8 Bake uncovered for 1 hour and 20 minutes, basting occasionally with juices from the bottom of the pan keep chicken moist.

Storage: Store in fridge for up to 1 week or in freezer for up to 3 months.

NUTRITION

Calories **624**
Total Fat **41g**
Saturated Fat **10g**
Unsaturated Fat **15g**
Cholesterol **214mg**
Sodium **241mg**
Carbohydrate **14g**
Dietary Fibre **3g**
Sugar **3g**
Protein **51g**

These pan-fried pork chops are **coated in a glossy apple glaze and seared to perfection** with the sweet autumn flavours of apple and cinnamon.

Apple Glazed **Pork Chops**

 YIELD: **4 PORK CHOPS**   SERVING SIZE: **1 PORK CHOP**   PREP TIME: **10 MINUTES**   COOK TIME: **20 MINUTES**

INGREDIENTS

- 350ml (12fl oz) unsweetened apple juice
- 50ml (2fl oz) pure maple syrup
- 2 tbsp Worcestershire Sauce
- ⅛ tsp cinnamon
- 4 x 110g (4oz) pork chops, bone in, with fat
- ⅛ tsp sea salt
- 1 tbsp olive oil
- 1 apple, cored and chopped
- 1 tsp fresh thyme, chopped

SPECIAL TOOLS

 MEAT THERMOMETER

METHOD

1 To make the apple glaze, combine the apple juice, maple syrup, Worcestershire Sauce, and cinnamon in a small saucepan. Bring contents to the boil. Reduce heat, cover, and simmer for 10 minutes. Remove from heat and set aside.

2 Heat olive oil in a frying pan over a medium-high heat. Season both sides of pork chops with sea salt. Add pork chops and spoon 125ml (4 fl oz) apple glaze on top.

3 Cook pork chops for 5 minutes per side or until internal temperature reaches 65°C (145°F), spooning sauce over pork chops occasionally to prevent pan from burning. Remove pork chops from heat and set aside.

4 Add chopped apple to pan with remaining sauce. Bring contents to the boil. Reduce heat and simmer for 10 minutes or until sauce has reduced by at least half.

5 Place pork chops on serving platter, top with apple and sauce mixture, and garnish with fresh thyme.

Storage: Pork chops can be refrigerated for up to 4 days.

NUTRITION

Calories 300	Saturated Fat 2g	Cholesterol 78mg	Carbohydrate 31g	Sugar 29g
Total Fat 8g	Unsaturated Fat 2g	Sodium 331mg	Dietary Fibre 1g	Protein 26g

This AIP version of the classic Catalan romesco sauce features **savoury garlic and sweet carrots,** which pair nicely with the spiciness of rocket.

Pork Tenderloin
with Roasted Carrot Romesco

 YIELD: **8 X 55G SLICES**   SERVING SIZE: **2 SLICES**   PREP TIME: **10 MINUTES**   COOK TIME: **20 MINUTES**

INGREDIENTS

680g (1½ lb) small carrots, peeled and halved lengthwise

3 tbsp olive oil

¼ tsp sea salt

450g (1lb) boneless pork tenderloin

1 clove garlic, peeled

2 tbsp red wine vinegar

450g (1lb) rocket

SPECIAL TOOLS

 OVENPROOF FRYING PAN

 MEAT THERMOMETER

 FOOD PROCESSOR

METHOD

1 Preheat oven to 230°C (450°F/ Gas 8). Line a baking tray with foil.

2 Toss carrots with 1 tablespoon olive oil and ⅛ teaspoon sea salt. Lay carrots on baking tray and roast for 15 to 20 minutes, turning occasionally until soft. Remove pan from oven and set aside.

3 In a large, ovenproof frying pan, heat 1 tablespoon olive oil over a medium-high heat. Season pork with ⅛ teaspoon sea salt. Cook pork in pan, turning occasionally, for 10 to 15 minutes, until golden brown on all sides.

4 Transfer frying pan to oven and cook for another 8 to 10 minutes or until the tenderloin reaches 65°C (145°F). Remove pan from oven, cover, and let sit for 5 minutes before slicing.

5 In a food processor, combine 1 tablespoon olive oil, garlic, 1 tablespoon red wine vinegar, 1 tablespoon water, and ⅓ of the roasted carrots. Process until smooth.

6 In a large bowl, toss the rocket with the remaining 1 tablespoon red wine vinegar.

7 Arrange remaining carrots and rocket on a serving platter. Top with sliced pork tenderloin and drizzle with carrot romesco sauce.

Storage: Tenderloin is best served immediately, but can be refrigerated for up to 4 days.

NUTRITION

| Calories 317 | Saturated Fat 4g | Cholesterol 75mg | Carbohydrate 17g | Sugar 8g |
| Total Fat 17g | Unsaturated Fat 12g | Sodium 249mg | Dietary Fiber 5g | Protein 25g |

These beef and bacon meatloaf muffins are **packed with plenty of nutritious veggies** and topped with a creamy sweet potato purée.

Meatloaf **Muffins**

 YIELD: **12 MUFFINS**   SERVING SIZE: **2 MUFFINS**   PREP TIME: **10 MINUTES**   COOK TIME: **20 MINUTES**

INGREDIENTS

2 tbsp olive oil

300g (10½ oz) onion, chopped

2 celery stalks, chopped

2 carrots, peeled and chopped

4 cloves garlic, minced

1 tsp marjoram

1 tsp dried basil

1 tsp dried oregano

¾ tsp sea salt

450g (1lb) minced beef

2 tbsp coconut flour

2 tsp Worcestershire Sauce

6g parsley, chopped

3 slices raw bacon, thinly sliced

450g (1lb) sweet potato, peeled and chopped

2 tbsp light coconut milk

1 tbsp ghee

SPECIAL TOOLS

 FOOD PROCESSOR

 MEAT THERMOMETER

 12-CUP MUFFIN PAN

METHOD

1 Preheat oven to 190°C (375°F). Heat olive oil in a large frying pan over a medium-high heat. Add onion, celery, carrots, and 3 teaspoons minced garlic. Cook for 5 minutes.

2 Add marjoram, basil, oregano, and ½ teaspoon sea salt. Cook for another 2 minutes.

3 Transfer vegetables to a large bowl. Add beef, coconut flour, Worcestershire Sauce, and parsley. Mix to combine.

4 Distribute meat mixture among 12 cups of a muffin pan. Press meat into muffin tin and top with 2 to 3 pieces of sliced bacon.

5 Bake meatloaf muffins for 20 minutes or until internal temperature reaches 68°C (155°F).

6 To make sweet potato purée, cover chopped sweet potatoes with water in a small saucepan. Bring to a boil. Reduce heat, cover, and simmer for 10 minutes or until fork-tender. Drain sweet potatoes.

7 In a food processor, combine sweet potatoes, coconut milk, 1 clove garlic, remaining ¼ teaspoon sea salt, and ghee. Process for 30 seconds or until smooth.

8 Top meatloaf muffins with sweet potato purée before serving.

Storage: Meatloaf muffins can be refrigerated for up to one week or frozen for up to 3 months.

Serving Suggestion: Top meatloaf muffins with sweet potato topping and garnish with chopped cooked bacon and fresh chives. Serve with Triple-Berry Barbecue Sauce if desired.

NUTRITION

Calories **329**

Total Fat **21g**

Saturated Fat **8g**

Unsaturated Fat **5g**

Cholesterol **58mg**

Sodium **517mg**

Carbohydrate **20g**

Dietary Fibre **5g**

Sugar **5g**

Protein **17g**

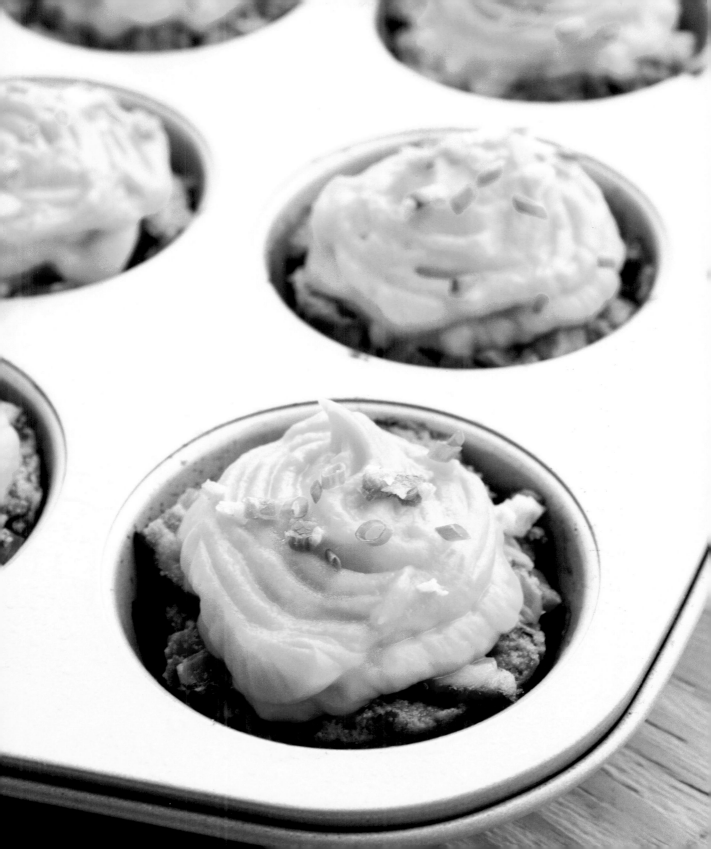

This blackened chicken has an enormous amount of flavour and **the perfect amount of char.** Use to top salads or mix into soups and stews.

Blackened Chicken Breast

 YIELD: **4 X 75G PIECES**   SERVING SIZE: **1 PIECE**   PREP TIME: **5 MINUTES**   COOK TIME: **6–10 MINUTES**

INGREDIENTS

450g (1lb) boneless, skinless chicken breast

1½ tsp dried oregano

1½ tsp dried thyme

1½ tsp garlic powder

1 tsp coconut sugar

½ tsp Seed-Free Curry Powder

¼ tsp sea salt

1 tbsp olive oil

METHOD

1 Rinse chicken breasts under cold water and place in a large zip-lock plastic bag. Using a meat tenderizer, pound meat into large, thin pieces.

2 On a large plate, combine oregano, thyme, garlic powder, coconut sugar, Seed-Free Curry Powder, and sea salt. Toss to mix.

3 Coat chicken breasts with spice mixture on both sides.

4 In a large frying pan or grill pan, heat olive oil over high heat.

5 Cook seasoned chicken in olive oil for 3 to 5 minutes on each side until chicken is blackened slightly on the outside and cooked through.

6 Remove chicken from pan and let sit for 5 minutes until cutting or serving.

Storage: Refrigerate chicken for up to 3 days or freeze for up to 3 months.

Serving Suggestion: Use for Grilled Chicken Cobb Salad or Caribbean Chicken Salad, or serve over a bed of fresh spinach with chopped strawberries.

NUTRITION

Calories **164**

Total Fat **4g**

Saturated Fat **0g**

Unsaturated Fat **3g**

Cholesterol **10mg**

Sodium **179mg**

Carbohydrate **3g**

Dietary Fibre **1g**

Sugar **1g**

Protein **26g**

Coated in **apricot preserves and shredded coconut,** these sweet chicken fingers are crispy on the outside and tender on the inside.

Crispy **Chicken Strips** with **Mango Honey Sauce**

 YIELD: **8 STRIPS**   SERVING SIZE: **2 STRIPS**   PREP TIME: **15 MINUTES**   COOK TIME: **25 MINUTES**

INGREDIENTS

- 450g (1lb) boneless, skinless chicken breast
- 2 tbsp coconut flour
- 2 tbsp arrowroot powder
- ½ tsp garlic powder
- ½ tsp onion powder
- ¼ tsp sea salt
- 125ml (4fl oz) light coconut milk
- 60g (2¼ oz) apricot preserves
- 60g (2¼ oz) unsweetened shredded coconut
- ½ tsp Seed-Free Curry Powder
- 1 cup mango, peeled and chopped
- 1 spring onion, chopped
- 1 clove garlic, peeled
- 1 tbsp honey
- 1 tbsp cider vinegar
- 1 tbsp lime juice

SPECIAL TOOLS

 FOOD PROCESSOR

METHOD

1 Preheat oven to 200°C (400°F/Gas 6). Line a baking tray with foil.

2 Rinse chicken breasts under cold water and place in large zip-lock plastic bag. Using a meat tenderizer, pound meat into large thin pieces. Remove chicken from bag and cut into 8 thin strips.

3 On a large plate, combine coconut flour, arrowroot powder, garlic powder, onion powder, and ⅛ tsp sea salt.

4 In a small bowl, whisk together coconut milk and apricot preserves.

5 On a separate large plate, combine shredded coconut and Seed-Free Curry Powder.

6 Dredge each chicken strip in coconut flour mixture, dip in coconut milk mixture, and coat with the shredded coconut mixture. Place coated chicken strips on prepared baking sheet.

7 Bake for 15 minutes. Flip chicken strips and bake for another 15 minutes on the other side.

8 To make dipping sauce, combine mango, spring onion, garlic, honey, cider vinegar, lime juice, and remaining ⅛ tsp sea salt in a food processor. Process until smooth.

Storage: Crispy Chicken Strips are best enjoyed immediately.

Serving Suggestion: Serve with a side of Rosemary Sweet Potato Crisps or Sea Salt Kale Crisps. Chicken strips can also be cut up and tossed on a salad.

NUTRITION

Calories **376**
Total Fat **11g**
Saturated Fat **8g**
Unsaturated Fat **0g**
Cholesterol **10mg**
Sodium **91mg**
Carbohydrate **39g**
Dietary Fibre **9g**
Sugar **22g**
Protein **30g**

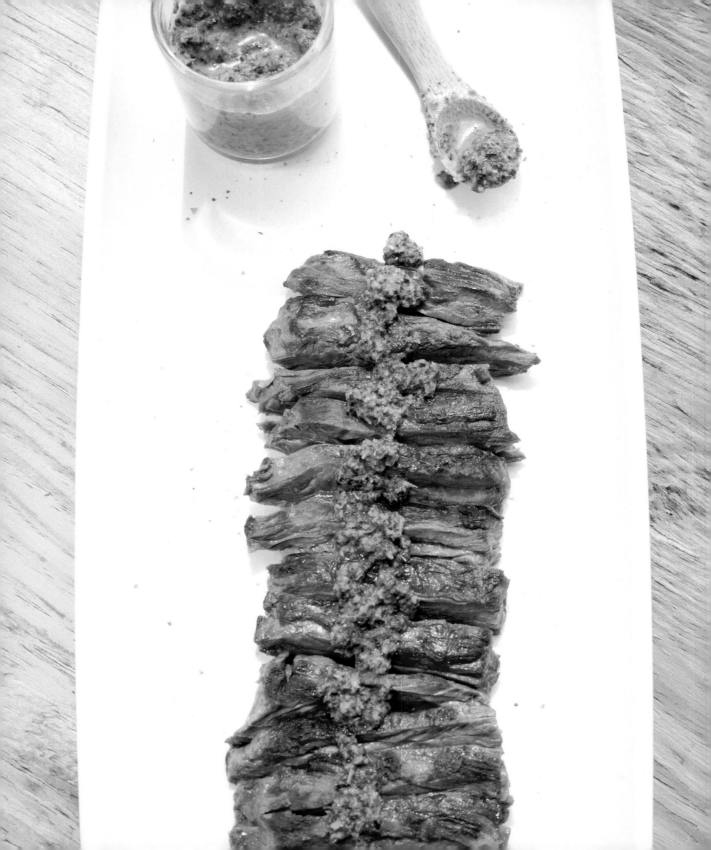

In Argentina, chimichurri sauce is served on grilled meats to add a burst of flavour. This **zesty, tangy sauce** is made with fresh herbs, garlic, and vinegar.

Chimichurri Skirt Steak

 YIELD: **4 X 75G PIECES**   SERVING SIZE: **1 PIECE**   PREP TIME: **10 MINUTES**   COOK TIME: **5 MINUTES**

INGREDIENTS

450g (1lb) skirt steak

50g (2oz) parsley, loosely packed

1 tsp sea salt

2 tbsp dried oregano

3 tbsp lemon juice

3 tbsp olive oil

3 tbsp sherry vinegar

5 cloves garlic, peeled

½ shallot, peeled

SPECIAL TOOLS

 FOOD PROCESSOR

METHOD

1 Remove steak from fridge and allow it to come to room temperature.

2 Meanwhile, in a food processor, combine parsley, sea salt, oregano, lemon juice, olive oil, sherry vinegar, garlic, and shallot. Process for 30 seconds or until chimichurri is well combined.

3 Heat frying pan over a medium-high heat. Rinse steak, pat dry, and spinkle with a pinch of salt on both sides.

4 Cook steak for 3 minutes of each side until seared and brown.

5 Remove steak from pan, cover with foil and let sit 5 minutes before cutting.

6 Cut steak into thin slices and top with chimichurri sauce.

Storage: Steak is best enjoyed immediately. Chimichurri can be made ahead of time and refrigerated for up to 3 days.

Serving Suggestion: Serve with a warm side dish such as Garlic Caper Roasted Cauliflower or Savoury Baked Butternut Squash.

NUTRITION

Calories **298**	Saturated Fat **5g**	Cholesterol **65mg**	Carbohydrate **6g**	Sugar **1g**
Total Fat **20g**	Unsaturated Fat **9g**	Sodium **675mg**	Dietary Fibre **2g**	Protein **25g**

An **overnight marinade of red wine and beef stock** infuses these lamb kebabs with savoury, succulent flavour.

Burgundy **Lamb Kebabs**

 YIELD: **4 KEBABS**   SERVING SIZE: **1 KEBAB**   PREP TIME: **5 MINUTES**   COOK TIME: **6 TO 10 MINUTES**

INGREDIENTS

450g (1lb) lamb stewing meat

2 cloves garlic, minced

1½ tbsp dried parsley

2 tsp olive oil

225ml (8fl oz) red wine

225ml (8fl oz) beef stock

¼ tsp sea salt

½ tsp lemon zest

1 large red onion

SPECIAL TOOLS

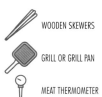

WOODEN SKEWERS

GRILL OR GRILL PAN

MEAT THERMOMETER

METHOD

1 In a large zip-lock bag, combine lamb, garlic, parsley, olive oil, red wine, beef stock, sea salt, and lemon zest. Marinate 8 to 10 hours or overnight.

2 Place 4 wooden skewers in a shallow pan of water to soak for 30 minutes. Preheat grill to high heat.

3 Cut onion into large pieces. Remove skewers from soaking water.

4 Assemble kebabs by threading marinated lamb pieces and onions alternately onto each skewer. Reserve the excess meat marinade.

5 Cook the skewers on the grill for 6 to 10 minutes, turning occasionally, and brushing with reserved marinade as needed. Cook lamb until meat reaches 68°C (155°F).

Storage: Store leftover kabobs in the fridge for up to 4 days.

Serving Suggestion: Serve Burgundy Lamb Kebabs over a bed of lettuce and top with Greek Red Wine Vinaigrette for a quick and easy Greek salad.

Cooking these kebabs over high heat allows for most of the alcohol in the wine of the marinade to cook off before consuming.

NUTRITION

Calories **225**

Total Fat **8g**

Saturated Fat **3g**

Unsaturated Fat **2g**

Cholesterol **74mg**

Sodium **225mg**

Carbohydrate **3g**

Dietary Fibre **0g**

Sugar **1g**

Protein **24g**

This recipe takes ribs from the grill to the slow cooker, with **sweet and smoky barbecue flavour** you can enjoy all year round.

Triple-Berry **Barbecued Ribs**

 YIELD: **24 RIBS** 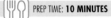 SERVING SIZE: **3 RIBS**   PREP TIME: **10 MINUTES** COOK TIME: **7 HOURS**

INGREDIENTS

1½ racks of ribs (about 1.5kg [3lb] total)

½ tsp sea salt

225ml (8fl oz) Triple-Berry Barbecue Sauce

SPECIAL TOOLS

 SLOW COOKER

METHOD

1 Cut each rack of ribs into smaller portions and season both sides with salt.

2 Brush ribs liberally with barbecue sauce and place in slow cooker, stacking them like shingles, one on top of the other.

3 Cook on high for 7 hours. Meat should be tender and falling off the bones.

Storage: Store leftover ribs in the fridge for up to 4 days.

Serving Suggestion: Serve ribs with additional barbecue sauce and a side of Honey Vinegar Tri-Coloured Coleslaw.

NUTRITION

Calories **465**

Total Fat **33g**

Saturated Fat **11g**

Unsaturated Fat **19g**

Cholesterol **118mg**

Sodium **801mg**

Carbohydrate **11g**

Dietary Fibre **1g**

Sugar **8g**

Protein **30g**

This salmon dinner is coated in a **simple homemade teriyaki sauce** made with all AIP-friendly ingredients.

Pineapple **Teriyaki Salmon**

 YIELD: **4 X 75G PIECES** SERVING SIZE: **1 PIECE** PREP TIME: **5 MINUTES** COOK TIME: **20 MINUTES**

INGREDIENTS

1 tbsp coconut oil

2 cloves garlic, minced

125ml (4fl oz) coconut aminos

1 tbsp honey

½ tsp fish sauce

1 tsp arrowroot powder

400g (14oz) pineapple, chopped

450g (1lb) salmon, bones removed and skin on

METHOD

1 Preheat oven to 180°C (350°F/Gas 4).

2 In a small saucepan over a medium-high heat, combine coconut oil and garlic. Stir to combine and cook for 2 minutes or until fragrant.

3 Reduce heat to medium-low and add coconut aminos, honey, and fish sauce.

4 Gradually whisk in arrowroot powder until sauce thickens. Remove from heat, cover, and set aside.

5 Line a baking dish with foil. Place pineapple at the bottom of the pan. Place salmon on top of pineapple and spoon sauce over the fish.

6 Bake for 15 minutes or until fish is flaky and pineapple is soft and caramelized.

Storage: Salmon is best served immediately, but leftovers can be refrigerated and used for lunch or dinner the following day.

Serving Suggestion: Serve salmon and grilled pineapple over Cauliflower Fried Rice.

Optional

Remove pineapple from the baking dish and transfer to a large frying pan or grill over high heat. Cook for 5 to 10 minutes or until pineapple begins to char.

NUTRITION

Calories **221**

Total Fat **8g**

Saturated Fat **4g**

Unsaturated Fat **26g**

Cholesterol **26mg**

Sodium **1,002mg**

Carbohydrate **15g**

Dietary Fibre **1g**

Sugar **11g**

Protein **21g**

A **sweet and savoury glaze** gives this baked salmon a delicious mouthful of flavour in every bite.

Maple Balsamic **Glazed Salmon**

 YIELD: **4 X 75G PIECES**   SERVING SIZE: **1 PIECE**   PREP TIME: **5 MINUTES**   COOK TIME: **15 MINUTES**

INGREDIENTS

450g (1lb) salmon, skin on, cut into 4 pieces

50ml (2fl oz) maple syrup

50ml (2fl oz) balsamic vinegar

2 cloves garlic, minced

1 tbsp olive oil

1 tbsp molasses

⅛ tsp sea salt

METHOD

1 Preheat oven to 220°C (425°F/Gas 7).

2 Line a baking tray with foil. Place salmon on baking sheet, skin-side down.

3 In a small bowl, whisk together maple syrup, balsamic vinegar, garlic, olive oil, molasses, and salt.

4 Brush salmon with glaze, reserving any excess. Bake 5 minutes, brush with more glaze, and return to oven. Repeat twice more, baking salmon for a total of 15 minutes.

5 Allow salmon to cool on the tray for a few minutes before serving. Lift the flesh from the skin to serve (the skin will stick to the foil). Discard the skin and foil.

Storage: Salmon can be stored in the fridge for up to 3 days.

Serving Suggestion: Serve salmon alongside a Classic Kale Salad.

NUTRITION

Calories **245**
Total Fat **7g**
Saturated Fat **1g**
Unsaturated Fat **6g**
Cholesterol **59mg**
Sodium **142mg**
Carbohydrate **20g**
Dietary Fibre **0g**
Sugar **20g**
Protein **23g**

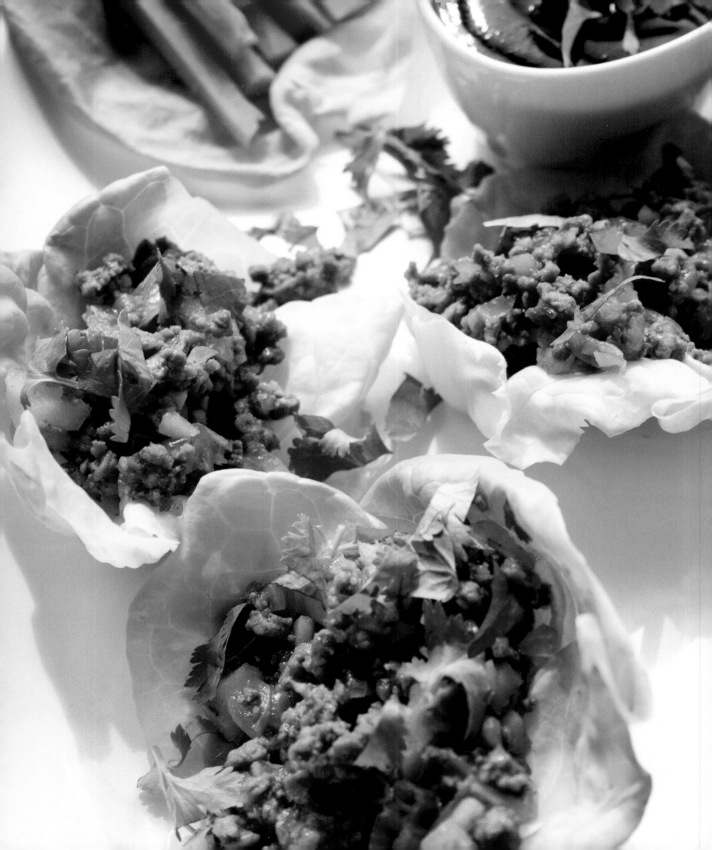

Dried plums, vinegar, and coconut aminos create a **tangy, sweet-and-salty plum sauce** perfect for dipping or drizzling over these healthy lettuce wraps.

Asian Turkey **Lettuce Wraps**

 YIELD: **16 WRAPS**   SERVING SIZE: **4 WRAPS**   PREP TIME: **10 MINUTES**   COOK TIME: **30 MINUTES**

INGREDIENTS

- 10 prunes, pitted
- 2 tbsp red onion, diced
- 3 tbsp coconut aminos
- 1 tbsp honey
- 1½ tsp cider vinegar
- 3 cloves minced garlic
- ⅛ tsp sea salt
- 225ml (8fl oz) water
- 450g (1lb) minced turkey (preferably dark meat)
- 1 large onion, chopped
- 1 tbsp fresh ginger, peeled and minced
- 113g (4oz) canned water chestnuts, drained and chopped
- 50g (2oz) spring onions, chopped
- 16 large butterhead lettuce leaves (about 2 heads lettuce)

METHOD

1. In a small saucepan over a medium-high heat, combine prunes, red onion, 1 tablespoon coconut aminos, honey, cider vinegar, 1 teaspoon minced garlic, salt, and water.

2. Bring contents to the boil, cover, and reduce heat to low. Simmer for 20 minutes.

3. Remove sauce from the heat and transfer to blender. Blend until smooth and set aside.

4. In a large frying pan over a medium-high heat, combine minced turkey, onion, remaining minced garlic, and ginger. Cook for 5 to 10 minutes or until meat is browned and onions are translucent and soft.

5. Add half the plum sauce and remaining 2 tablespoons coconut aminos to turkey mixture. Cook for another 5 minutes.

6. Remove pan from heat and stir in water chestnuts and spring onions.

7. Spoon 2 tablespoons turkey mixture into each lettuce leaf. Drizzle with remaining plum sauce.

Storage: Lettuce wraps are best enjoyed immediately, but the turkey mixture can be refrigerated for up to 4 days.

Serving Suggestion: Top lettuce wraps with chopped cucumber, shredded carrots, and fresh coriander if desired.

SPECIAL TOOLS

 BLENDER

NUTRITION

Calories **333**
Total Fat **14g**
Saturated Fat **4g**
Unsaturated Fat **0g**
Cholesterol **85mg**
Sodium **398mg**
Carbohydrate **32g**
Dietary Fibre **4g**
Sugar **15g**
Protein **20g**

Roasting this **delicate white fish with lemon and herbs** is a quick and easy way to bring out its mild, subtle flavour.

Lemon-Stuffed **Sea Bass**

 YIELD: **2 FISH**   SERVING SIZE: **1 FISH**   PREP TIME: **10 MINUTES**   COOK TIME: **20 MINUTES**

INGREDIENTS

2 whole sea bass, cleaned with gills and fins removed (about 1kg; 2lb)

2 tbsp olive oil

2 cloves garlic, thinly sliced

1 lemon, sliced

4 sprigs rosemary

4 sprigs thyme

4 sprigs parsley

125ml (4fl oz) dry white wine

⅛ tsp sea salt

METHOD

1 Preheat oven to 240°C (475°F/Gas 9).

2 Rub fish with 1 tablespoon olive oil on all sides.

3 Stuff each fish cavity with half of the garlic slices, 3 lemon slices, and 2 sprigs each of rosemary, thyme, and parsley.

4 Drizzle remaining 1 tablespoon olive oil into baking pan and place fish on top. Pour half the wine over the fish and sprinkle with sea salt.

5 Bake for 10 minutes. Flip fish, pour remaining white wine over fish, and bake for another 10 minutes.

6 Remove from oven and squeeze remaining lemon slices over fish before serving.

Storage: Sea bass is best served immediately.

NUTRITION

Calories 456	Saturated Fat 2g	Cholesterol 29mg	Carbohydrate 5g	Sugar 1g
Total Fat 16g	Unsaturated Fat 11g	Sodium 177mg	Dietary Fibre 1g	Protein 54g

A zesty coconut milk sauce unites the flavours of tender, **sweet scallops and crispy, salty bacon** in this decadent dish.

Bacon-Wrapped **Scallops**

 YIELD: **12 SCALLOPS**   SERVING SIZE: **3 SCALLOPS**   PREP TIME: **10 MINUTES**   COOK TIME: **12 MINUTES**

INGREDIENTS

450g (1 lb) large sea scallops

12 slices of bacon

50ml (2fl oz) light coconut milk

Juice of 1 lime

2 tbsp fresh coriander, chopped

METHOD

1 Preheat grill. Line a baking dish with foil.

2 Rinse scallops under cold water and pat dry with kitchen paper.

3 Roll each scallop in a slice of bacon and secure with a cocktail stick.

4 Place scallops in baking dish and grill for 6 minutes.

5 Flip scallops and grill for another 6 minutes until tops are golden brown and scallops are cooked through.

6 In a small bowl, whisk together coconut milk, lime juice, and coriander.

7 Drizzle cooked scallops with coconut milk mixture before serving.

Storage: Scallops are best served immediately.

NUTRITION

| Calories 300 | Saturated Fat 6g | Cholesterol 72mg | Carbohydrate 7g | Sugar 2g |
| Total Fat 16g | Unsaturated Fat 0g | Sodium 1,169mg | Dietary Fibre 0g | Protein 32g |

Indulge in the **rich, gamey flavour of duck** paired with **savoury leeks, chewy figs,** and a **sticky honey glaze**.

Roast Duck with Shallots, Figs, and Honey

 YIELD: **800G**   SERVING SIZE: **200G**   PREP TIME: **15 MINUTES**   COOK TIME: **1 HOUR**

INGREDIENTS

- 2 x 225g (½ lb) duck breasts, skin on
- ⅛ tsp sea salt
- 3 tsp fresh thyme, chopped
- 2 tbsp olive oil
- 2 large leeks, white and green parts, thinly sliced
- 4 carrots, peeled and chopped
- 2 tbsp honey
- 125ml (4fl oz) plus 1 tsp red wine
- 55g (2oz) pancetta, chopped
- 150g (5½oz) dried figs, chopped and stems removed
- 125ml (4fl oz) vegetable stock

SPECIAL TOOLS

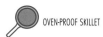 OVEN-PROOF SKILLET

METHOD

1 Preheat oven to 180°C (350°F/ Gas 4). Rinse duck breasts under cold water and pat dry with kitchen paper. With a sharp knife, score the fat of the duck breast in a crisscross pattern. Season duck breasts with salt and 2 teaspoons thyme.

2 In a large ovenproof frying pan, heat olive oil over a medium-high heat. Add leeks and carrots. Cook for 20 minutes or until vegetables are soft.

3 Push vegetables to the side and place duck breasts, skin-side down, in the centre of the pan. Cook, undisturbed, for 10 minutes.

4 In a small bowl, whisk together honey and 1 teaspoon red wine. Flip duck breasts and brush with honey mixture.

5 Transfer frying pan to the oven and roast for 10 minutes. Brush duck breasts with remaining honey mixture and roast for another 10 minutes or until internal temperature reaches 74°C (165°F).

6 In a saucepan over a medium-high heat, cook pancetta for 3 minutes or until crispy. Add figs, remaining red wine, vegetable stock, and remaining 1 teaspoon thyme. Bring contents to the boil, reduce heat, and simmer for 10 minutes.

7 Remove frying pan from oven and let sit for 5 minutes. Top with fig sauce before serving.

Storage: Duck is best served immediately.

NUTRITION

| Calories 577 | Saturated Fat 6g | Cholesterol 10mg | Carbohydrate 53g | Sugar 33g |
| Total Fat 25g | Unsaturated Fat 14g | Sodium 356mg | Dietary Fibre 7g | Protein 37g |

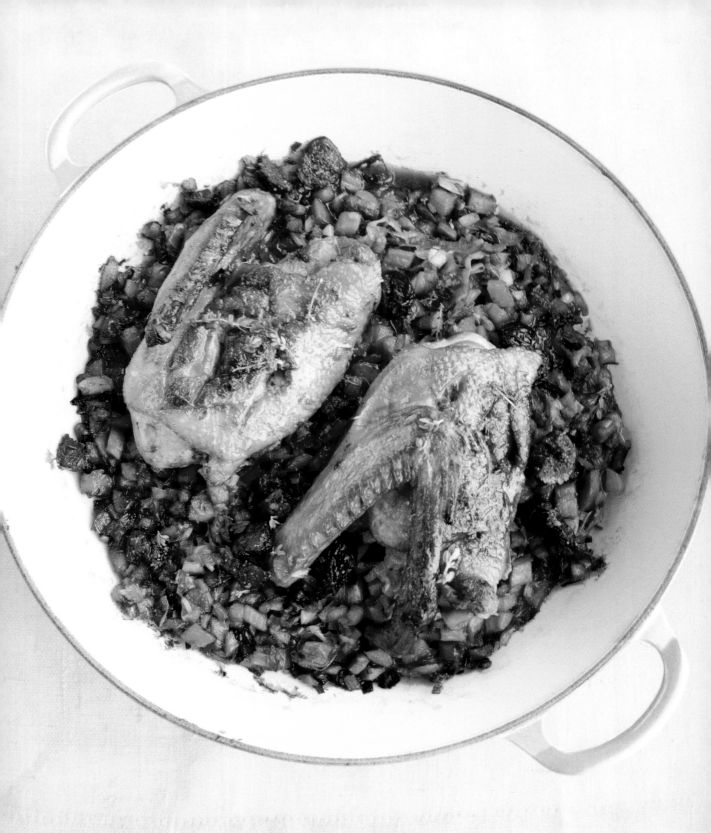

The simple ingredients of onion, garlic, and orange come together to create a **juicy pulled pork with a tangy citrus flavor**.

Orange Pulled Pork **Carnitas**

 YIELD: **2KG (4½ LB)** SERVING SIZE: **300G (10 OZ)** PREP TIME: **15 MINUTES** COOK TIME: **8 HOURS**

INGREDIENTS

1.6kg (3½lb) boneless pork shoulder

2 TB. olive oil

¼ tsp. sea salt

1 TB. dried oregano

1½ tsp. Seed-Free Curry Powder

300g (10oz) red onion, thinly sliced (1 large onion)

5 cloves garlic, sliced

1 orange, halved

SPECIAL TOOLS

 SLOW COOKER

METHOD

1 Rinse pork shoulder under cold water and pat dry with paper towels.

2 In a small bowl, combine olive oil, salt, oregano, and Seed-Free Curry Powder. Rub mixture on all sides of pork shoulder.

3 Place pork shoulder in slow cooker. Add onions and garlic to slow cooker, on top of the pork shoulder.

4 Squeeze the orange over the vegetables and meat and toss the remainder of the orange into the slow cooker. Cover and cook on low for 8 hours.

5 Remove meat from slow cooker and place on cutting board. Let meat cool slightly and pull it apart using two forks to shred it.

Storage: Refrigerate for 5 days or freeze for up to 3 months.

Serving Suggestion: Top carnitas with chopped coriander, white onion, and avocado to add Mexican flair, or add Triple-Berry Barbecue Sauce for a smoky summer dish.

NUTRITION

| Calories 541 | Saturated Fat 13g | Cholesterol 141mg | Carbohydrate 4g | Sugar 2g |
| Total Fat 39g | Unsaturated Fat 22g | Sodium 230mg | Dietary Fiber 1g | Protein 35g |

These burgers feature lean bison and are spiced with the robust **Mediterranean** flavours of garlic and curry.

Middle Eastern **Bison Burgers**

 YIELD: **4 PATTIES** 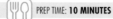 SERVING SIZE: **1 PATTY** PREP TIME: **10 MINUTES** 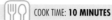 COOK TIME: **10 MINUTES**

INGREDIENTS

450g (1lb) minced bison

75g (2½oz) red onion, chopped (¼ large onion)

5g (⅛oz) parsley, chopped

2 cloves garlic, minced

2 tsp Seed-Free Curry Powder

1 tsp salt

1 tbsp olive oil

METHOD

1 In a large bowl, combine minced bison, red onion, parsley, garlic, Seed-Free Curry Powder, and salt.

2 With clean hands, mix ingredients until well combined and form into 4 tightly packed hamburger patties.

3 In a large frying pan, heat olive oil over medium-high heat. Add burger patties and cook, undisturbed, for 4 minutes.

4 Flip burgers and cook for another 4 minutes on the other side.

Storage: Refrigerate for 5 days or freeze for up to 3 months.

Serving Suggestion: Serve over a bed of lettuce with a side of Rosemary Sweet Potato Chips.

NUTRITION

Calories **291**	Saturated Fat **8g**	Cholesterol **79mg**	Carbohydrate **2g**	Sugar **0g**
Total Fat **22g**	Unsaturated Fat **11g**	Sodium **660mg**	Dietary Fiber **0g**	Protein **22g**

The **mild, sweet flavour and noodle-like texture** of spaghetti squash makes it an ideal substitute for traditional pasta noodles.

Herbed Baked
Spaghetti Squash

 YIELD: **775G**   SERVING SIZE: **195G**   PREP TIME: **5 MINUTES**   COOK TIME: **45 MINUTES**

INGREDIENTS

1 medium spaghetti squash (about 2kg [4lb])

2 tbsp olive oil

1 tbsp fresh rosemary, chopped

1 tbsp fresh thyme, chopped

⅛ tsp sea salt

METHOD

1 Preheat oven to 200°C (400°F/Gas 6). Line a baking tray with foil.

2 Cut spaghetti squash lengthways. Scoop out and discard seeds.

3 Place squash halves on baking tray, flesh-side up. Drizzle each half with olive oil, massaging the oil into the flesh to ensure it is well coated.

4 Sprinkle rosemary, thyme, and sea salt over the squash halves.

5 Bake for 30 to 45 minutes or until squash is fork tender.

6 Remove squash from oven and let cool for 10 to 20 minutes. Using a fork, carefully scrape the squash out of the skin.

Storage: Spaghetti squash can be stored in the fridge for up to 4 day.

Serving Suggestion: Serve spaghetti squash with Tomato-Less Pasta Sauce or Pork and Fennel Meatballs.

NUTRITION

Calories **100**

Total Fat **8g**

Saturated Fat **1g**

Unsaturated Fat **6g**

Cholesterol **0mg**

Sodium **80mg**

Carbohydrate **9g**

Dietary Fibre **2g**

Sugar **4g**

Protein **1g**

This nontraditional pasta dish features **crunchy, spiralized courgette 'noodles'** coated in a creamy pesto sauce made with garlic and basil.

Garlic Pesto
Courgette Pasta

 YIELD: **ABOUT 2KG**   SERVING SIZE: **250G**   PREP TIME: **10 MINUTES**   COOK TIME: **3 MINUTES**

INGREDIENTS

1 tbsp plus175ml (6fl oz) olive oil

8 medium courgettes, spiralized

50g (2oz) fresh basil leaves

1 avocado, pit and skin removed

3 tbsp lemon juice

3 cloves garlic, peeled

⅛ tsp dried oregano

⅛ tsp dried thyme

Dash sea salt

SPECIAL TOOLS

 SPIRALIZER

 FOOD PROCESSOR

METHOD

1 In a large frying pan, heat 1 tablespoon olive oil over a medium-high heat until hot. Add courgette noodles and toss for 2 to 3 minutes until slightly tender. Remove from pan and set aside.

2 In a food processor, combine basil, avocado, lemon juice, remaining olive oil, garlic, oregano, thyme, and sea salt. Process for 30 seconds or until smooth.

3 In a large bowl, toss courgette noodles with avocado pesto.

Storage: Courgette pasta is best enjoyed immediately. Pesto can be stored in an airtight container in the fridge for up to 3 days.

A spiralizer tool turns vegetables into faux noodles. Whether you're making courgette noodles, potato spirals, or swede pasta, a spiralizer is an inexpensive way to create versatile, AIP-friendly noodles.

NUTRITION

Calories **237**

Total Fat **25g**

Saturated Fat **3g**

Unsaturated Fat **18g**

Cholesterol **0mg**

Sodium **18mg**

Carbohydrate **5g**

Dietary Fibre **2g**

Sugar **3g**

Protein **2g**

In this recipe, **carrots, broccoli, and courgette** take the place of traditional noodles, while tangy fish sauce and vinegar **mimic classic pad thai** flavour.

Pad Thai Noodles

 YIELD: **ABOUT 900G**   SERVING SIZE: **300G**   PREP TIME: **15 MINUTES**   COOK TIME: **10 MINUTES**

INGREDIENTS

- 4 medium carrots, peeled
- 1 medium courgette, peeled
- 2 tbsp coconut oil
- 3 cloves garlic, minced
- 50ml (2fl oz) fish sauce
- 2 tbsp coconut aminos
- 50ml (2fl oz) lime juice
- 1 tbsp cider vinegar
- 255g (9oz) broccoli slaw
- 115g (4oz) spring onions, chopped
- 15g (½oz) fresh coriander, chopped
- 1 lime, cut into wedges

METHOD

1 Using a vegetable peeler, create carrot and courgette 'noodles' by shaving the vegetables in long, thin strokes.

2 In a large frying pan, combine coconut oil and garlic. Sauté for 2 minutes or until soft.

3 Add fish sauce, coconut aminos, lime juice, and cider vinegar. Simmer for 5 minutes or until sauce is reduced by half.

4 Add carrots, courgette, broccoli slaw, and spring onions. Toss to coat and cook for 2 to 3 minutes.

5 Remove pan from heat and top with coriander and lime wedges.

Storage: Pad Thai Noodles are best served immediately.

Serving Suggestion: Top noodles with your choice of cooked chicken or shrimp.

Preshredded broccoli slaw can be found near the bagged lettuce in some supermarkets. Its sturdy, crunchy texture makes an excellent stand-in for noodles in stir-fries.

NUTRITION

Calories **199**	Saturated Fat **9g**	Cholesterol **0mg**	Carbohydrate **17g**	Sugar **8g**
Total Fat **10g**	Unsaturated Fat **0g**	Sodium **2,301mg**	Dietary Fibre **6g**	Protein **11g**

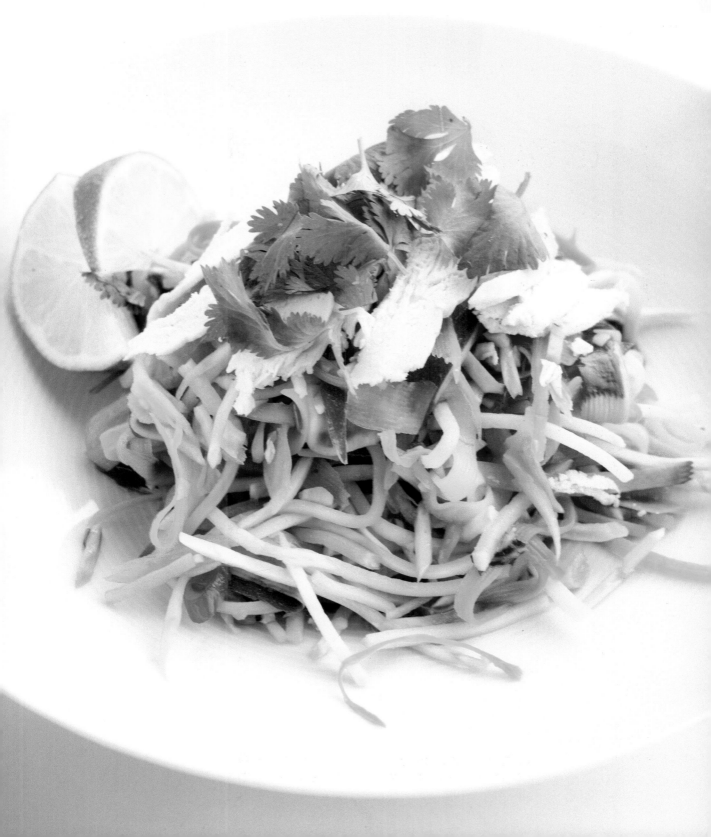

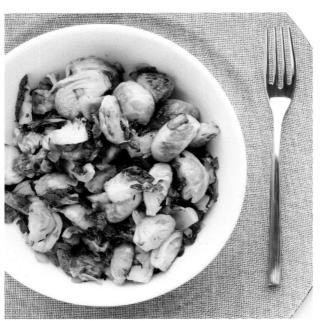
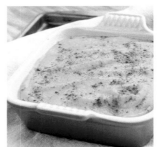
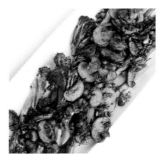

CHAPTER 6
Side Dishes

In this warm side dish, the **nuttiness of roasted cauliflower** is enhanced by the **zesty, briny flavours** of lemon and capers.

Garlic Caper
Roasted Cauliflower

 YIELD: **650G**　　 SERVING SIZE: **325G**　　 PREP TIME: **10 MINUTES**　　 COOK TIME: **25 MINUTES**

INGREDIENTS

1 meduium head cauliflower, cut into florets

1 tbsp coconut oil, melted

2 tbsp olive oil

6g fresh parsley, chopped

1 tbsp lemon zest

50ml (2 fl oz) lemon juice

2 tbsp non-pareil capers, chopped

1 clove garlic, minced

METHOD

1 Preheat oven to 200°C (400°F/Gas 6). Line a baking tray with foil.

2 Spread cauliflower on baking tray and drizzle with coconut oil, massaging it into the florets to ensure they are well coated.

3 Roast cauliflower for 15 minutes. Flip cauliflower pieces and roast for another 10 minutes or until edges are crisp and golden brown.

4 In a small bowl, combine olive oil, parsley, lemon zest, lemon juice, capers, and garlic. Whisk to combine.

5 In a large bowl, toss roasted cauliflower with dressing before serving.

Storage: Cauliflower is best enjoyed immediately, but can be refrigerated for up to 48 hours.

Serving Suggestion: Serve cauliflower as a savoury side dish to Chimichurri Skirt Steak or Blackened Chicken Breast.

NUTRITION

Calories 269	Saturated Fat 8g	Cholesterol 0mg	Carbohydrate 19g	Sugar 8g
Total Fat 21g	Unsaturated Fat 12g	Sodium 92mg	Dietary Fibre 8g	Protein 6g

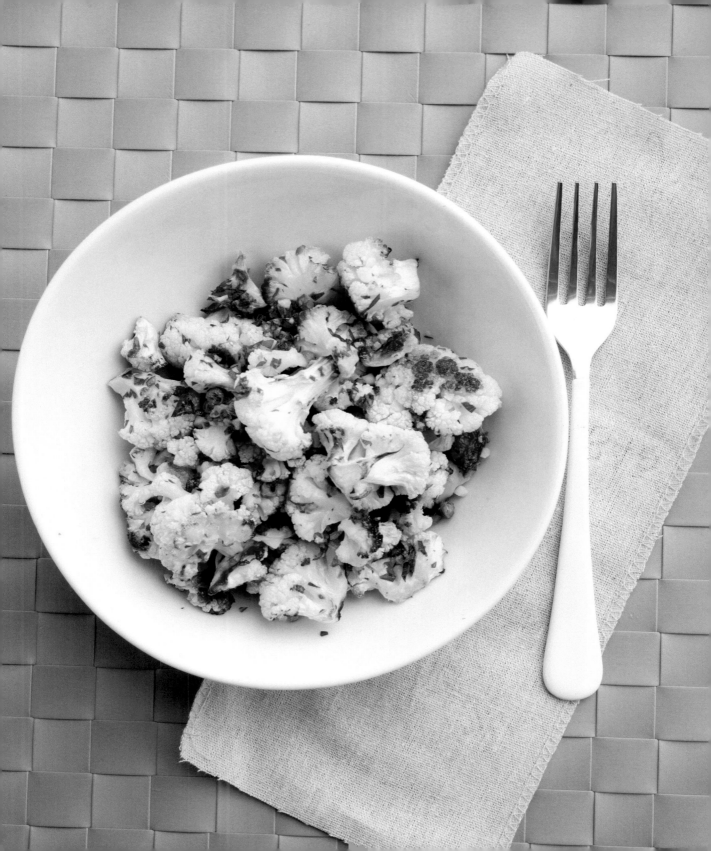

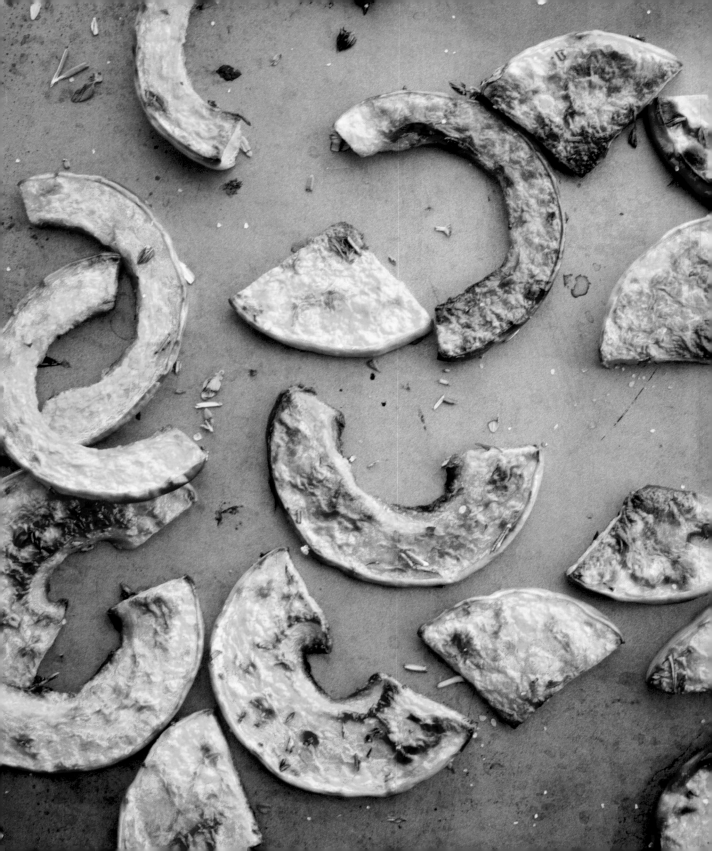

This quick and satisfying side dish features **butternut squash and savoury fresh herbs** roasted until tender and golden brown.

Savoury Baked
Butternut Squash

 YIELD: **ABOUT 800G**   SERVING SIZE: **200G**   PREP TIME: **5 MINUTES**   PREP TIME: **5 MINUTES** COOK TIME: **20 MINUTES**

INGREDIENTS

1 butternut squash, sliced
and seeds removed

1 tbsp olive oil

½ tsp fresh rosemary, chopped

½ tsp fresh thyme, chopped

Pinch sea salt

METHOD

1 Preheat oven to 200°C (400°F/Gas 6). Line a baking tray with foil.

2 Place squash on baking tray and drizzle with olive oil, massaging it into the squash with clean hands to ensure it is well coated.

3 Sprinkle squash with rosemary, thyme, and sea salt.

4 Roast squash for 10 minutes. Flip and roast for another 10 minutes until squash is golden brown and fork-tender.

Storage: Squash can be refrigerated for up to 4 days.

Serving Suggestion: Serve squash as a savoury side dish to Chimichurri Skirt Steak or Apple Glazed Pork Chops.

Butternut squash is usually prepared by removing and discarding the thin, beige skin. However, the skin softens when roasted and is, in fact, edible.

NUTRITION

| Calories 93 | Saturated Fat 0g | Cholesterol 0mg | Carbohydrate 16g | Sugar 3g |
| Total Fat 4g | Unsaturated Fat 3g | Sodium 44mg | Dietary Fibre 3g | Protein 1g |

Roasting green beans in balsamic vinegar gives this **crunchy side dish** a **delicious tangy bite.**

Roasted Balsamic **Green Beans**

 YIELD: **450G**   SERVING SIZE: **115G**   PREP TIME: **5 MINUTE**   COOK TIME: **10 MINUTES**

INGREDIENTS

450g (1lb) green beans, ends trimmed and discarded

1 tbsp olive oil

4 tsp balsamic vinegar

Pinch sea salt

METHOD

1 Preheat oven to 200°C (400°F). Line a baking tray with foil.

2 Place green beans on baking tray. Drizzle with olive oil and 3 teaspoons balsamic vinegar.

3 Massage the oil and vinegar into the green beans with clean hands. Sprinkle with sea salt.

4 Roast green beans for 10 minutes or until tender.

5 Remove pan from oven and toss green beans with remaining 1 teaspoon balsamic vinegar before serving.

Storage: Green beans can be stored in the fridge for up to 3 days.

NUTRITION

| Calories 60 | Saturated Fat 0g | Cholesterol 0mg | Carbohydrate 6g | Sugar 3g |
| Total Fat 3g | Unsaturated Fat 2g | Sodium 31mg | Dietary Fibre 2g | Protein 1g |

This cranberry relish is packed with nutrient-dense wholefoods, including **tart cranberries, chewy sultanas,** and **crunchy apples.**

Orange Cranberry **Relish**

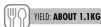 YIELD: **ABOUT 1.1KG**   SERVING SIZE: **120G**   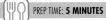 PREP TIME: **5 MINUTES**   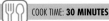 COOK TIME: **30 MINUTES**

INGREDIENTS

400g (14oz) whole cranberries

175ml (6fl oz) maple syrup

75g (2¾ oz) sultanas

2 tsp ground cinnamon

1 tsp ground ginger

225ml (8fl oz) water

half an onion, chopped

1 medium apple, peeled and chopped

225ml (8fl oz) orange juice

METHOD

1 In a medium saucepan, combine cranberries, maple syrup, sultanas, cinnamon, ginger, and water.

2 Heat over a medium-high heat, uncovered, for 15 minutes or until the cranberries have popped and begin to soften.

3 Add onion, apple, and orange juice. Continue cooking, uncovered, for another 15 minutes until mixture has thickened.

Storage: Cranberry relish can be refrigerated for up to 1 week or frozen for up to 3 months.

NUTRITION

Calories **225**	Saturated Fat **0g**	Cholesterol **0mg**	Carbohydrate **58g**	Sugar **45g**
Total Fat **0g**	Unsaturated Fat **0g**	Sodium **7mg**	Dietary Fibre **6g**	Protein **1g**

Pan-searing Brussels sprouts in **rich and flavourful** bacon fat renders them tender and delicious, with **crispy, caramelized outer leaves**.

Pan-Seared **Brussels Sprouts** with Bacon

| 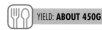 YIELD: **ABOUT 450G** | SERVING SIZE: **75G** | PREP TIME: **10 MINUTES** | COOK TIME: **25 MINUTES** |

INGREDIENTS

4 slices bacon, chopped

450g (1lb) Brussels sprouts, trimmed and quartered

half a large onion, chopped

METHOD

1 In a large frying pan, cook bacon over a medium-high heat for 5 minutes or until crispy.

2 Remove bacon from pan and place on a clean plate lined with kitchen paper to absorb excess grease.

3 In remaining bacon fat, cook onion and Brussels sprouts for 15 to 20 minutes or until tender and caramelized.

4 Remove pan from heat and stir bacon into Brussels sprouts mixture.

Storage: These Brussels sprouts are best served immediately, but can be stored in the refrigerator for up to 2 days.

Serving Suggestion: Serve as a side dish with Lemon-Stuffed Sea Bass.

NUTRITION

| Calories 60 | Saturated Fat 1g | Cholesterol 3mg | Carbohydrate 7g | Sugar 2g |
| Total Fat 3g | Unsaturated Fat 0g | Sodium 109mg | Dietary Fibre 3g | Protein 4g |

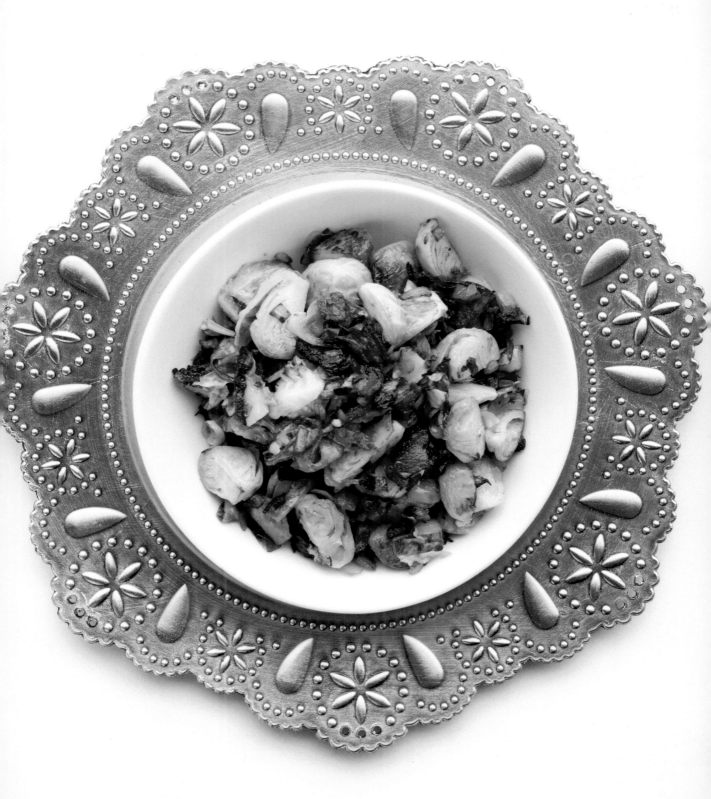

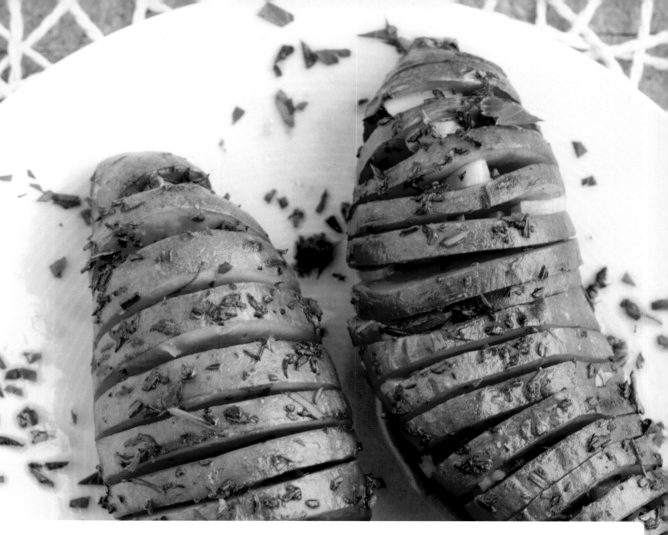

How to Hasselback

The potatoes in this dish are cut in a style called 'Hasselback', named for the Swedish restaurant where the technique originated. The thin slices not only look impressive, but provide pockets for flavourful additions like garlic, ghee, and fresh herbs. Although it appears complex, it's easy to prepare.

1 Using a sharp knife, slice a portion of the potato flesh from the base of the potato to create a flat, even surface for the potato to sit on.

2 Slice the potatoes the short way, creating cuts about 3mm (⅛-inch) apart, making sure not to cut entirely through the potato and stopping about 6mm (¼ inch) from the bottom.

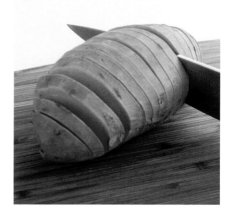

Swap traditional baked potatoes for these accordion-sliced sweet potatoes, which are **crisp on the outside** and **soft and tender on the inside**.

Hasselback **Sweet Potatoes**

 YIELD: 4 POTATOES   **SERVING SIZE: 1 POTATO**   **PREP TIME: 10 MINUTES**   **COOK TIME: 50 MINUTES**

INGREDIENTS

- 4 medium sweet potatoes
- 4 garlic cloves, thinly sliced
- 3 tbsp ghee, melted
- 1 tbsp fresh rosemary, finely chopped
- 1 tbsp fresh sage, finely chopped
- ¼ tsp salt

METHOD

1 Preheat oven to 190°C (375°F/Gas 5).

2 Hasselback the potatoes and press a piece of sliced garlic into each of the potato grooves.

3 Place potatoes in a baking dish. Brush with melted ghee and sprinkle with rosemary, sage, and salt. Cover pan with foil.

4 Bake for 50 minutes or until potatoes are fork-tender.

5 Remove dish from oven and spoon juices from the bottom of the dish over the potatoes before serving.

Storage: Sweet potatoes are best served straight from the oven, but can be refrigerated for up to 2 days.

Serving Suggestion: Serve alongside Greek-Style Roast Chicken or Blackened Chicken Breast.

Variation: To make Cinnamon Hasselback Sweet Potatoes, replace the garlic slices with thinly sliced apples, use ground cinnamon instead of sage, and drizzle potatoes with honey instead of ghee before baking.

NUTRITION

Calories **194**
Total Fat **10g**
Saturated Fat **6g**
Unsaturated Fat **3g**
Cholesterol **25mg**
Sodium **187mg**
Carbohydrate **25g**
Dietary Fibre **4g**
Sugar **7g**
Protein **3g**

Grated cauliflower mimics the texture of rice in this **salty, savoury stand-in** for the **Chinese take-away favourite**.

Cauliflower **Fried Rice**

 YIELD: **ABOUT 1KG**   SERVING SIZE: **250G**   PREP TIME: **5 MINUTES**   COOK TIME: **15 MINUTES**

INGREDIENTS

1 medium head cauliflower, cut into florets

1 tbsp olive oil

150g (5½oz) onion, chopped

150g (5½oz) carrots, chopped

1 tbsp fresh ginger, peeled and minced

1 clove garlic, minced

3 spring onions, chopped

1 tbsp coconut aminos

1 tbsp Worcestershire Sauce

SPECIAL TOOLS

 FOOD PROCESSOR

METHOD

1 In a food processor fitted with a chopping blade, pulse cauliflower for 5 to 10 seconds or until it is finely grated and resembles rice.

2 In a large frying pan over high heat, add olive oil, onion, carrots, ginger, and garlic. Cook for 5 minutes or until soft.

3 Add cauliflower, stir, and cook for 5 minutes undisturbed, allowing the cauliflower to brown. Stir contents, scraping any browned bits from the bottom, and cook for another 5 minutes undisturbed.

4 Remove pan from heat. Stir in spring onions, coconut aminos, and Worcestershire Sauce until the 'rice' is evenly coated.

Storage: Cauliflower rice is best served immediately.

Serving Suggestion: Serve as side dish with Broccoli Beef Stir-Fry or Pineapple Teriyaki Salmon.

Use a hot, dry pan. Let the cauliflower brown at the bottom of the pan to prevent it from releasing too much liquid, which can cause the 'rice' to become mushy.

NUTRITION

Calories **105**	Saturated Fat **1g**	Cholesterol **0mg**	Carbohydrate **17g**	Sugar **7g**
Total Fat **4g**	Unsaturated Fat **4g**	Sodium **189mg**	Dietary Fibre **5g**	Protein **3g**

The **creamy texture** of this easy-to-prepare side dish makes it the perfect healthy, AIP-friendly **substitute for traditional mashed potatoes**.

Parsnip Purée

 YIELD: **300G**   SERVING SIZE: **75G**   PREP TIME: **5 MINUTES** COOK TIME: **30 MINUTES**

INGREDIENTS

- 300g (10½ oz) parsnips, peeled and chopped
- 1 clove garlic, peeled
- 2 tbsp ghee
- 50ml (2 fl oz) light coconut milk
- ¼ tsp smoked sea salt

SPECIAL TOOLS

 FOOD PROCESSOR

METHOD

1 In a medium saucepan, cover parsnips and garlic with water. Cover and boil for 20 minutes over high heat.

2 Drain the parsnips, reserving the cooking liquid.

3 In a food processor, combine cooked parsnips, garlic, ghee, coconut milk, 50ml (2 fl oz) reserved cooking liquid, and smoked sea salt. Process for 30 seconds or until smooth.

Storage: Store in the fridge for up to 1 week or in the freezer for up to 3 months.

Serving Suggestion: Serve as a warm side dish with Apple Glazed Pork Chops or Meatloaf Muffins.

Variation: To make Swede Purée, substitute the same amount of swede for the parsnips.

NUTRITION

Calories **234**	Saturated Fat **10g**	Cholesterol **33mg**	Carbohydrate **25g**	Sugar **7g**
Total Fat **15g**	Unsaturated Fat **5g**	Sodium **304mg**	Dietary Fibre **6g**	Protein **2g**

The lightly sweet, earthy flavour of butternut squash is complemented by **creamy coconut milk and maple syrup** in this hearty side dish.

Coconut **Butternut Squash** Mash

 YIELD: ABOUT 1.3KG   **SERVING SIZE: 225G**   PREP TIME: **10 MINUTES**   COOK TIME: **40 MINUTES**

INGREDIENTS

1 medium butternut squash, cut in half lengthways and seeds removed

3 tbsp ghee

50ml (2fl oz) light coconut milk

2 tbsp plus 1 tsp maple syrup

¼ tsp sea salt

⅛ tsp cinnamon

SPECIAL TOOLS

 FOOD PROCESSOR

METHOD

1 Preheat oven to 190°C (375°F/Gas 5).

2 Line a baking tray with foil. Place butternut squash halves flesh-side down. Bake for 30 to 40 minutes or until fork tender.

3 Scoop butternut squash out of the skin and put in a food processor.

4 Add ghee, coconut milk, maple syrup, and sea salt. Process for 30 seconds or until smooth.

5 Scoop into a serving dish and sprinkle with cinnamon.

Storage: Store in the fridge for up to 3 days or freeze for up to 3 months.

Variation: To make Maple Sweet Potato Mash, replace butternut squash with 600g (1lb 5oz) peeled and chopped sweet potatoes.

NUTRITION

Calories 124	Saturated Fat 4g	Cholesterol 17mg	Carbohydrate 16g	Sugar 7g
Total Fat 7g	Unsaturated Fat 2g	Sodium 86mg	Dietary Fibre 3g	Protein 1g

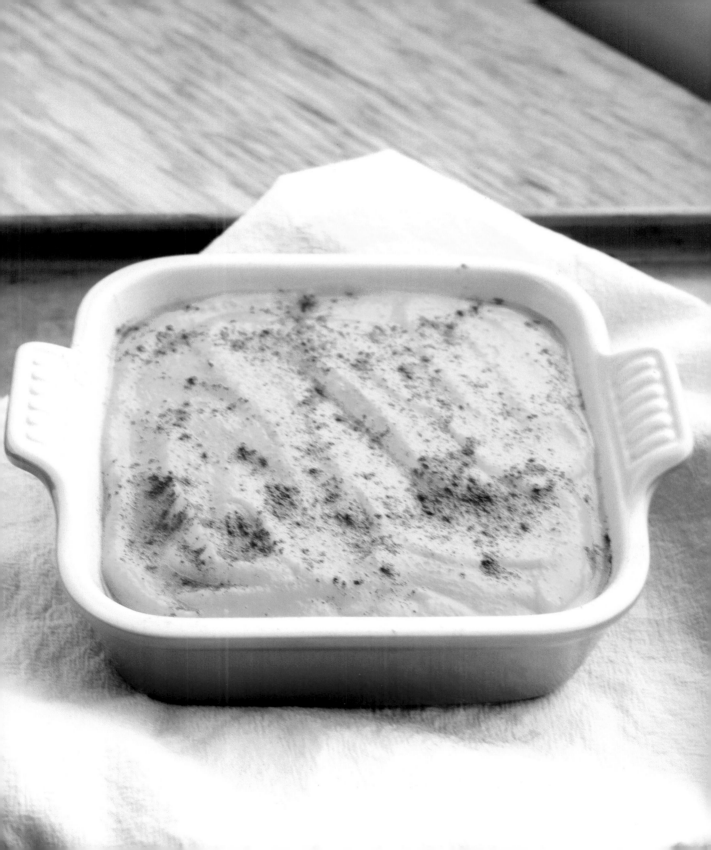

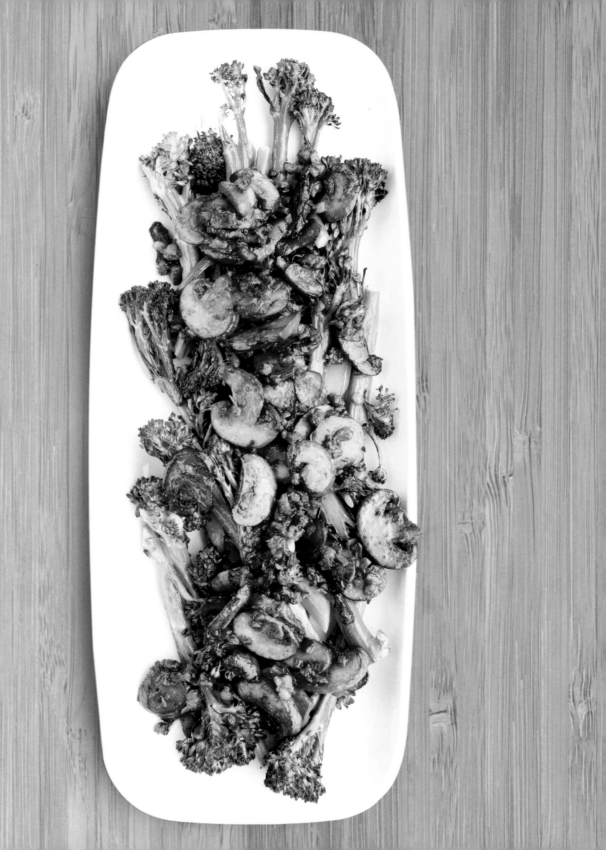

Tenderstem broccoli has a milder, more delicate flavour than broccoli. Here it is topped with the **smoky, savoury flavours of pancetta, mushrooms, and garlic.**

Roasted Tenderstem Broccoli
with White Wine Mushrooms

 YIELD: **700G**   SERVING SIZE: **175G**   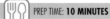 PREP TIME: **10 MINUTES**   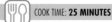 COOK TIME: **25 MINUTES**

INGREDIENTS

2 bunches tenderstem broccoli, leaves removed and ends trimmed

1 tbsp olive oil

1 tbsp bacon fat

35g (1¼ oz) shallots, chopped

1 clove garlic, minced

225g (8oz) cremini mushrooms, sliced

55g (2oz) pancetta, chopped

50ml (2 fl oz) dry white wine

METHOD

1 Preheat oven to 200°C (400°F/Gas 6). Line a baking tray with foil.

2 Place tenderstem broccoli on baking sheet. Drizzle with olive oil and massage oil into vegetables until well coated. Roast for 10 minutes.

3 In a large frying pan over a medium-high heat, combine the bacon fat, shallots, garlic, mushrooms, and pancetta. Sauté for 10 minutes or until vegetables are tender.

4 Deglaze pan with wine and allow alcohol to cook off for another 2 to 5 minutes.

5 Remove tenderstem broccoli from oven and transfer to a serving dish. Spoon white wine mushroom sauce over the tenderstem broccoli.

Storage: Tenderstem broccoli is best served immediately, but can be stored in the fridge for up to 3 days.

Serving Suggestion: Serve as a side dish with Lemon-Stuffed Sea Bass or Bacon-Wrapped Scallops.

NUTRITION

| Calories **196** | Saturated Fat **3g** | Cholesterol **13mg** | Carbohydrate **10g** | Sugar **2g** |
| Total Fat **13g** | Unsaturated Fat **5g** | Sodium **128mg** | Dietary Fibre **3g** | Protein **6g** |

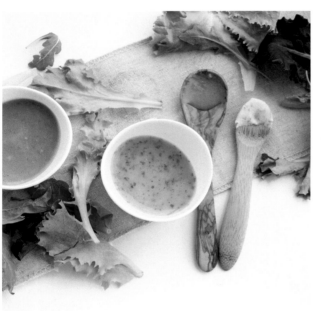

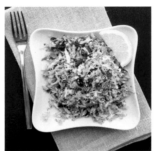

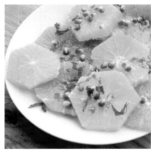

CHAPTER 7

Salads

& Dressings

Coriander Lime Vinaigrette

 YIELD: **225ML**   SERVING SIZE: **2 TBSP**   PREP TIME: **5 MINUTES**   COOK TIME: **0 MINUTES**

INGREDIENTS

1 clove garlic, peeled

3 tbsp lime juice

3 tbsp orange juice

2 tbsp honey

1 tsp fresh ginger,
  peeled and minced

1 tbsp fresh coriander, chopped

50ml (2fl oz) olive oil

⅛ tsp sea salt

METHOD

1 In a food processor, combine garlic, lime juice, orange juice, honey, ginger, coriander, olive oil, and sea salt.

2 Process for 30 seconds or until smooth. Transfer to an airtight container.

Storage: Store in an airtight container in the fridge for up to 1 week.

Serving Suggestion: Serve with Caribbean Chicken Salad or Citrus Mint Salad.

SPECIAL TOOLS

 FOOD PROCESSOR

NUTRITION

Calories **81**

Total Fat **7g**

Saturated Fat **1g**

Unsaturated Fat **6g**

Cholesterol **0mg**

Sodium **37mg**

Carbohydrate **6g**

Dietary Fibre **0g**

Sugar **5g**

Protein **0g**

Greek Red Wine Vinaigrette

 YIELD: **175ML**   SERVING SIZE: **2 TBSP**   PREP TIME: **5 MINUTES**   COOK TIME: **0 MINUTES**

INGREDIENTS

125ml (4fl oz) olive oil

2 tbsp lemon juice

2 tbsp red wine vinegar

1 clove garlic, peeled

1 tsp dried oregano

¼ tsp sea salt

METHOD

1 In a food processor, combine olive oil, lemon juice, red wine vinegar, garlic, oregano, and sea salt.

2 Process for 30 seconds or until smooth. Transfer to an airtight container.

Storage: Store in an airtight container or jar in the fridge for up to 1 week.

SPECIAL TOOLS

 FOOD PROCESSOR

NUTRITION

Calories **163**

Total Fat **18g**

Saturated Fat **2g**

Unsaturated Fat **15g**

Cholesterol **0mg**

Sodium **98mg**

Carbohydrate **1g**

Dietary Fibre **0g**

Sugar **0g**

Protein **0g**

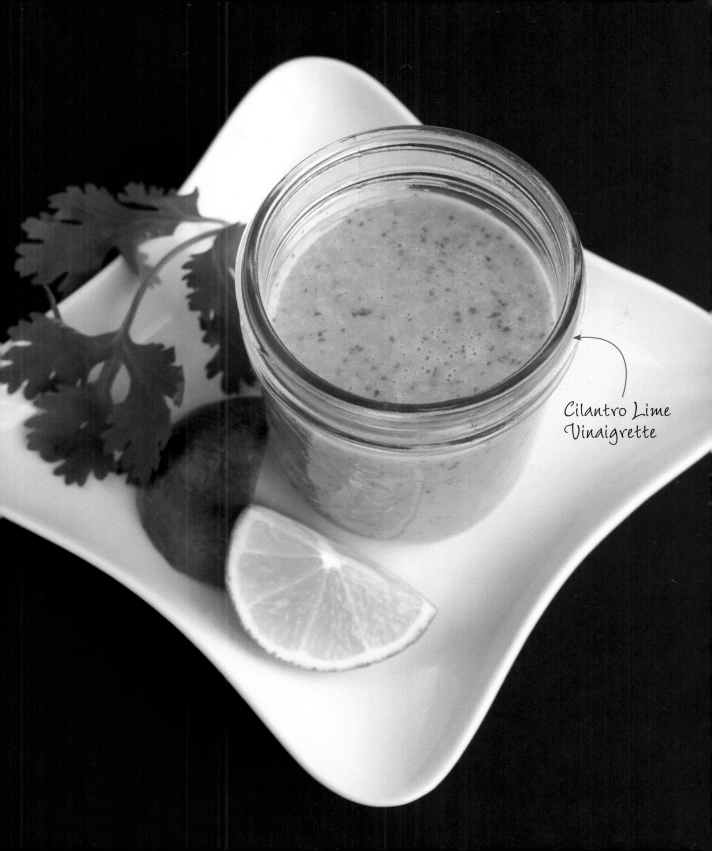

Cilantro Lime
Vinaigrette

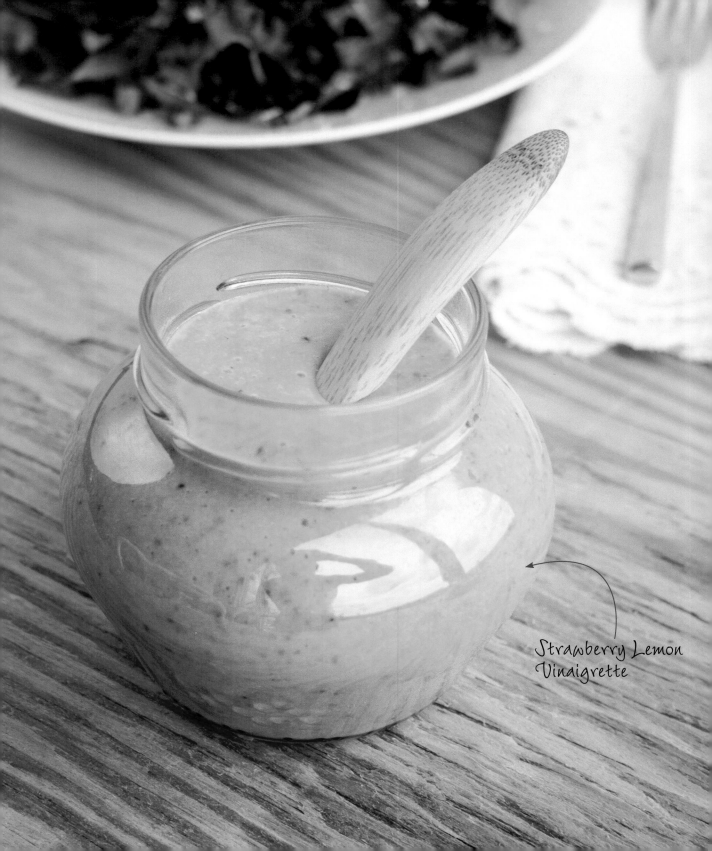

Strawberry Lemon
Vinaigrette

Strawberry Lemon Vinaigrette

 YIELD: **450ML**   SERVING SIZE: **2 TBSP**   PREP TIME: **5 MINUTES**   COOK TIME: **0 MINUTES**

INGREDIENTS

600g (1lb 5oz) strawberries, hulled

125ml (4 fl oz) olive oil

50ml (2 fl oz) orange juice

1 tbsp lemon juice

1 tbsp balsamic vinegar

2 cloves garlic, peeled

1 tsp lemon zest

⅛ tsp sea salt

SPECIAL TOOLS

 FOOD PROCESSOR

METHOD

1 In a food processor, combine strawberries, olive oil, orange juice, lemon juice, balsamic vinegar, garlic, lemon zest, and sea salt.

2 Process for 30 seconds or until smooth. Transfer to an airtight container.

Storage: Store in an airtight container or jar in the fridge for up to 1 week.

NUTRITION

Calories **73**
Total Fat **7g**
Saturated Fat **1g**
Unsaturated Fat **6g**
Cholesterol **0mg**
Sodium **16mg**
Carbohydrate **3g**
Dietary Fibre **1g**
Sugar **2g**
Protein **0g**

Carrot Ginger Dressing

 YIELD: **450ML**   SERVING SIZE: **2 TBSP**   PREP TIME: **5 MINUTES**   COOK TIME: **20 MINUTES**

INGREDIENTS

75g (2¾oz) carrot, peeled and chopped

125ml (4 fl oz) water

2 tbsp fresh ginger, minced

⅛ tsp sea salt

2 tbsp lemon juice

2 tbsp cider vinegar

2 tbsp honey

1 tbsp olive oil

3 tbsp light coconut milk

SPECIAL TOOLS

 FOOD PROCESSOR

METHOD

1 In a small saucepan, combine carrots and water. Bring to the boil. Reduce heat, cover, and simmer for 20 minutes or until fork-tender.

2 Transfer carrots and boiling water to food processor and add ginger, sea salt, lemon juice, cider vinegar, honey, olive oil, and coconut milk.

3 Process for 30 seconds or until smooth. Transfer to an airtight container.

Storage: Store in an airtight container or jar in the fridge for up to 1 week.

NUTRITION

Calories **20**
Total Fat **1g**
Saturated Fat **0g**
Unsaturated Fat **1g**
Cholesterol **0mg**
Sodium **18mg**
Carbohydrate **3g**
Dietary Fibre **0g**
Sugar **3g**
Protein **0g**

Celeriac, also known as celery root, has a **mild celery flavour** and crunchy texture that pairs well with **savoury herbs and a sweet citrus dressing**.

Apple Currant **Celeriac Slaw**

 YIELD: **ABOUT 800G**   SERVING SIZE: **200G**   PREP TIME: **10 MINUTES**   COOK TIME: **0 MINUTES**

INGREDIENTS

1 large bulb celeriac, peeled and quartered

1½ large apples, peeled and quartered

1 tbsp orange juice

Juice and zest of 1 lemon

⅛ tsp sea salt

1 tbsp fresh thyme, chopped

2 tbsp fresh basil, chopped

75g (2¾oz) dried currants, or raisins

SPECIAL TOOLS

 FOOD PROCESSOR

METHOD

1 Fit food processor with a shredding disc attachment. Feed celeriac and apple quarters into machine to grate.

2 In a small bowl, combine orange juice, lemon juice, lemon zest, and salt to make the dressing.

3 In a large bowl, combine grated celeriac and apple mixture with thyme, basil, and currants.

4 Pour dressing over slaw and toss to combine. Let sit for 5 minutes before serving.

Storage: Slaw is best enjoyed immediately.

Serving Suggestion: Serve as a side dish with Blackened Chicken Breast or Lemon-Stuffed Sea Bass.

Celeriac is a variety of celery cultivated for its edible root. This turnip-sized root has a knobbly outer surface and smooth, white flesh with a mild, celery-like flavour.

NUTRITION

| Calories 171 | Saturated Fat 0g | Cholesterol 0mg | Carbohydrate 42g | Sugar 25g |
| Total Fat 0g | Unsaturated Fat 0g | Sodium 231mg | Dietary Fibre 6g | Protein 3g |

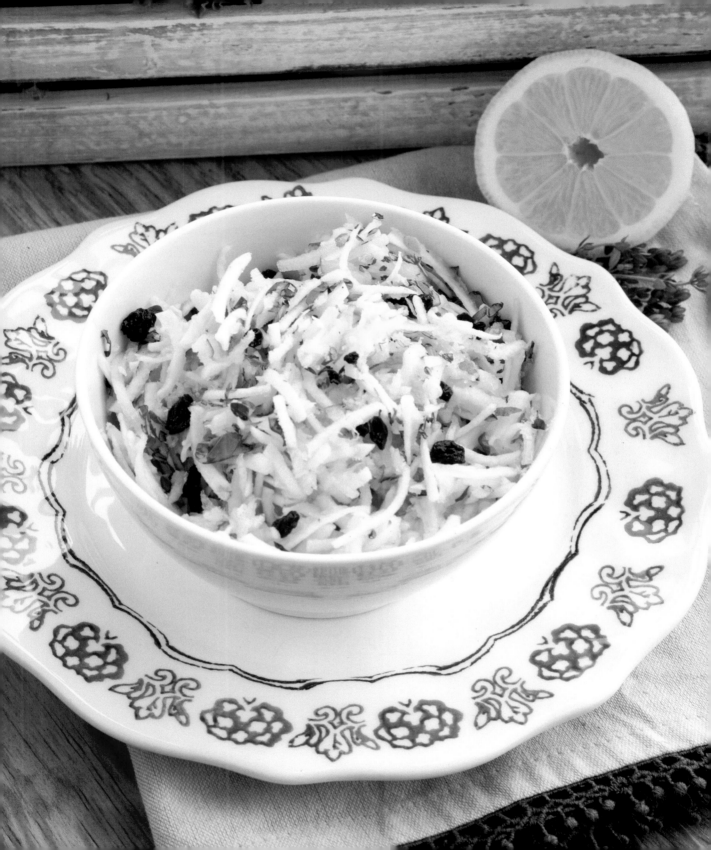

Put a **Mediterranean twist on a traditional favourite** with this unique tuna salad featuring plenty of crunchy, fresh vegetables and a **tangy avocado mayonnaise**.

Mediterranean **Tuna Salad**

 YIELD: **1.6KG**   SERVING SIZE: **200G**   PREP TIME: **15 MINUTES**   CHILL TIME: **15 MINUTES**

INGREDIENTS

4 x 170g cans albacore tuna, drained

1 x 395g can artichoke hearts, drained and chopped

50g (1¾oz) celery, chopped

75g (2¾oz) cucumber, chopped

140g (5oz) green olives, pitted and chopped

150g (5½oz) red onion, chopped

6g parsley, chopped

6g fresh basil, chopped

1 tsp dried oregano

115g Basic Avocado "Mayonnaise"

½ tsp sea salt

METHOD

1 In a large bowl, combine tuna, artichoke hearts, celery, cucumber, green olives, red onion, parsley, basil, oregano, Basic Avocado "Mayonnaise," and sea salt. Gently stir until well mixed.

2 Refrigerate salad for 15 minutes before serving to allow flavours to come together.

Storage: Salad can be stored in the fridge for up to 3 days.

Serving Suggestion: Serve over a bed of mixed greens or crunchy romaine lettuce.

NUTRITION

Calories 192	Saturated Fat 2g	Cholesterol 13mg	Carbohydrate 6g	Sugar 1g
Total Fat 10g	Unsaturated Fat 3g	Sodium 832mg	Dietary Fibre 3g	Protein 18g

Guacamole meets chicken salad in this creamy combination of avocado, shredded chicken, and crunchy cucumber.

Avocado **Chicken Salad**

 YIELD: **ABOUT 1.2KG**   SERVING SIZE: **200G**   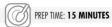 PREP TIME: **15 MINUTES**   CHILL TIME: **30 MINUTES**

INGREDIENTS

- 560g (1lb 4oz) cooked chicken breast, chopped
- 150g (5½oz) cucumber, finely chopped
- 150g (5½oz) red onion, finely chopped
- 1 clove garlic, minced
- Juice of 1½ limes
- 15g (½oz) fresh coriander, chopped
- 2 avocados, mashed
- ½ tsp sea salt

METHOD

1 In a large mixing bowl, combine chicken, cucumber, red onion, garlic, lime juice, fresh coriander, mashed avocado, and sea salt. Gently stir until well mixed.

2 Refrigerate salad for 30 minutes before serving to allow flavours to come together.

Storage: Salad can be stored in the fridge for up to 3 days.

Serving Suggestion: Serve salad over a bed of mixed greens, as a dip with chopped veggies, or alongside Rosemary Sweet Potato Crisps or Cinnamon Apple Crisps for a quick snack.

NUTRITION

Calories 283	Saturated Fat 2g	Cholesterol 79mg	Carbohydrate 7g	Sugar 2g
Total Fat 13g	Unsaturated Fat 2g	Sodium 221mg	Dietary Fibre 3g	Protein 38g

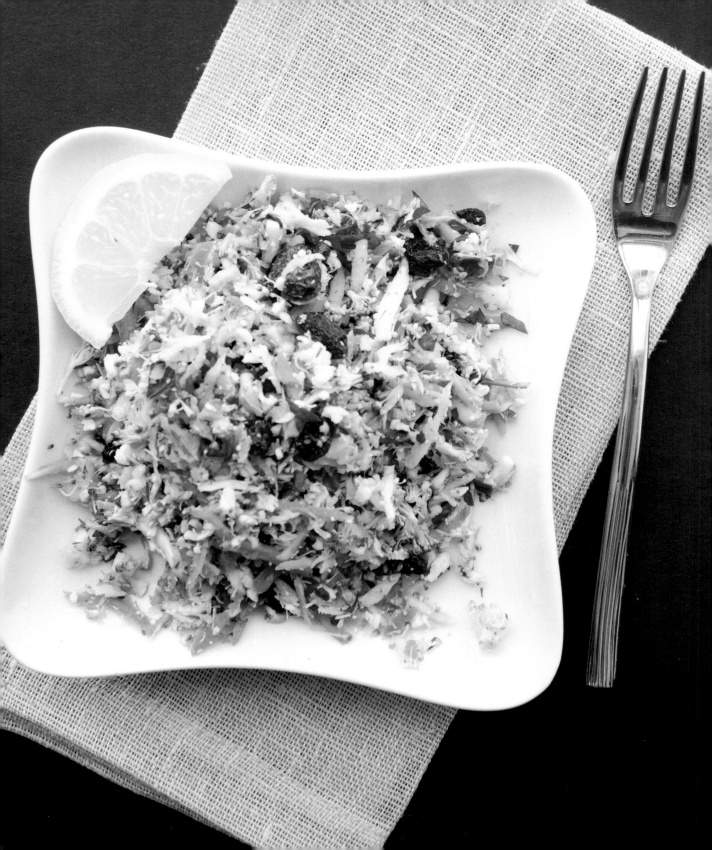

Cruciferous vegetables give this salad a **crunchy** texture, while the raisins and pineapple juice offer a **subtle hint of sweetness**.

Shaved **Broccoli and Cauliflower** Slaw

 YIELD: **2.9KG**   SERVING SIZE: **450G**   PREP TIME: **10 MINUTES**   CHILL TIME: **20 MINUTES**

INGREDIENTS

1.4kg (about 3 lb) broccoli florets

600g cauliflower florets

375g (13oz) carrots, peeled and roughly chopped

300g (10½oz) raisins

25g (1oz) parsley, chopped

125ml (4fl oz) lemon juice

125ml (4fl oz) pineapple juice

1 tbsp lemon zest

¼ tsp sea salt

SPECIAL TOOLS

 FOOD PROCESSOR

METHOD

1 Fit food processor with a shredding disk attachment. Feed broccoli into machine and pulse until finely shredded. Transfer to a large bowl.

2 Feed cauliflower into food processor to grate. Transfer to the large bowl with the broccoli.

3 Feed carrots into food processor, pulse until finely shredded, and add to bowl with broccoli and cauliflower. Stir to combine.

4 Add raisins and parsley to the vegetable mixture and stir to combine.

5 In a small bowl, whisk together lemon juice, pineapple juice, lemon zest, and salt. Pour dressing over slaw and toss to combine.

6 Refrigerate for 20 minutes before serving to allow for flavours to come together.

Storage: Slaw is best served immediately, but can be stored in the fridge for up to 2 days.

NUTRITION

Calories **274**	Saturated Fat **0g**	Cholesterol **0mg**	Carbohydrate **67g**	Sugar **42g**
Total Fat **1g**	Unsaturated Fat **0g**	Sodium **199mg**	Dietary Fibre **9g**	Protein **8g**

This summer salad offers the **fresh citrus flavours** of orange and grapefruit complemented by **tart pomegranate seeds** and **refreshing mint**.

Citrus Mint Salad

 YIELD: **ABOUT 900G**   SERVING SIZE: **225g**   PREP TIME: **5 MINUTES**   COOK TIME: **0 MINUTES**

INGREDIENTS

- 2 oranges, peeled and sliced
- 1 grapefruit, peeled and sliced
- 180g (6oz) pomegranate seeds
- 2 tbsp lime juice
- 2 tbsp honey
- 1 tbsp fresh mint leaves, chopped

METHOD

1 On large platter, arrange orange, grapefruit, and pomegranate seeds.

2 In a small bowl, whisk together lime juice and honey.

3 Drizzle dressing over fruit and garnish with mint leaves.

Storage: Salad can be refrigerated for up to 3 days.

To remove pomegranate seeds, cut the fruit into quarters, submerge in a bowl of water, and gently remove the seeds from the pith. The seeds will sink to the bottom and the pith will float to the top.

NUTRITION

| Calories 133 | Saturated Fat 0g | Cholesterol 0mg | Carbohydrate 33g | Sugar 23g |
| Total Fat 1g | Unsaturated Fat 0g | Sodium 3mg | Dietary Fibre 4g | Protein 2g |

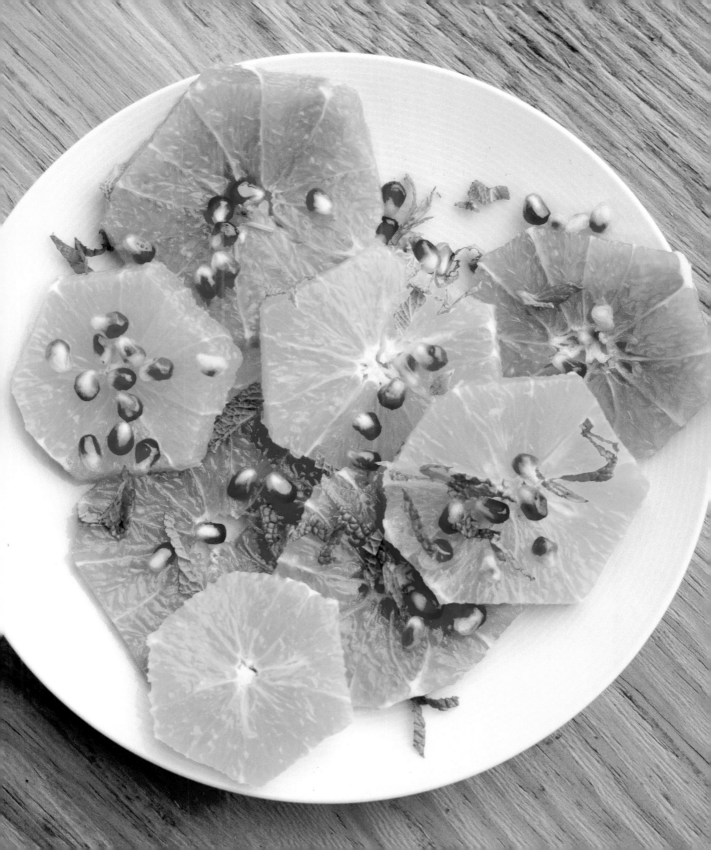

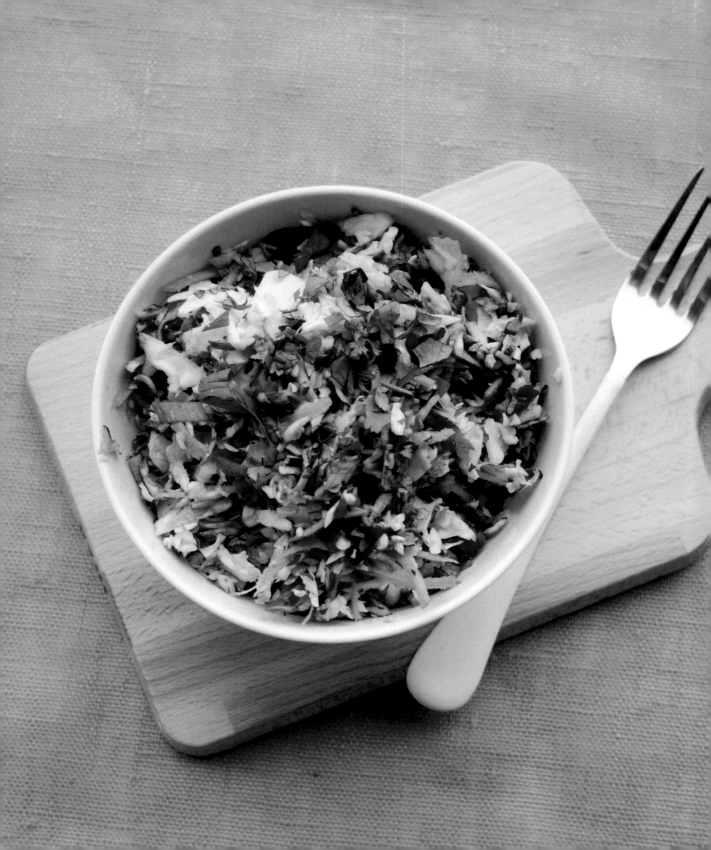

Vinegar-based slaws are lighter than traditional creamy ones. Packed with **tangy flavour**, this slaw makes a great side dish for any **summer barbecue**.

Honey Vinegar
Tri-Coloured Coleslaw

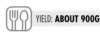 YIELD: **ABOUT 900G**　　 SERVING SIZE: **100G**　　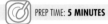 PREP TIME: **5 MINUTES**　　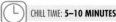 CHILL TIME: **5–10 MINUTES**

INGREDIENTS

300g (10½ oz) red cabbage, shredded

300g (10½ oz) green cabbage, shredded

2 carrots, peeled and shredded

50g (2oz) spring onions, chopped

2 tbsp cider vinegar

4 tbsp olive oil

1 clove garlic, minced

2 tbsp honey

¼ tsp sea salt

15g (½oz) fresh coriander, chopped

METHOD

1 In a large bowl, combine red cabbage, green cabbage, carrots, and spring onions.

2 In a small bowl, whisk together cider vinegar, olive oil, garlic, honey, and sea salt.

3 Pour dressing over cabbage mixture and toss to coat. Stir in fresh coriander.

4 Refrigerate for 5 to 10 minutes before serving to allow flavours to come together.

Storage: Slaw is best served immediately.

Serving Suggestion: Serve as a refreshing side dish with Pineapple Teriyaki Salmon or Middle Eastern Bison Burgers.

To quickly shred cabbage and carrots, use the shredding disk attachment that comes with most food processors. This attachment is often reversible to create fine or coarse shreds.

SPECIAL TOOLS

 FOOD PROCESSOR

NUTRITION

| Calories **109** | Saturated Fat **1g** | Cholesterol **0mg** | Carbohydrate **12g** | Sugar **8g** |
| Total Fat **6g** | Unsaturated Fat **0g** | Sodium **103mg** | Dietary Fibre **3g** | Protein **1g** |

Fresh flavours of lemon juice and garlic join with creamy butternut squash and bright cranberries to create the **perfect warm winter salad**.

Classic Kale Salad

 YIELD: **ABOUT 900G**   SERVING SIZE: **450G**   PREP TIME: **10 MINUTES**   COOK TIME: **20 MINUTES**

INGREDIENTS

400g (14oz) butternut squash, peeled and cubed

1 tbsp olive oil

⅛ tsp sea salt

550g (1lb 4oz) kale, stems removed and roughly chopped

2 tbsp lemon juice

2 tbsp Greek Red Wine Vinaigrette

1 tbsp honey

30g (1oz) dried cranberries

METHOD

1 Preheat oven to 190°C (375°F/Gas 5).

2 Line a baking tray with foil. Spread butternut squash on baking tray, drizzle with olive oil, and sprinkle with sea salt. Bake for 10 minutes.

3 While squash bakes, combine kale, lemon juice, and Greek Red Wine Vinaigrette in a large bowl. Using clean hands, massage dressing into kale leaves.

4 Remove squash from the oven. Turn over the pieces and bake for another 5 minutes.

5 Remove squash from the oven, drizzle with honey, and bake for another 5 minutes.

6 Add squash and dried cranberries to kale and toss until combined.

Storage: Refrigerate for up to 2 days.

Serving Suggestion: Top warm kale salad with Greek-Style Roast Chicken, Maple Balsamic Glazed Salmon, or Lemon-Stuffed Sea Bass.

> Massaging the lemon juice and dressing into the kale tenderizes the tough greens and minimizes the natural bitter flavours.

NUTRITION

| Calories **218** | Saturated Fat **1g** | Cholesterol **0mg** | Carbohydrate **35g** | Sugar **13g** |
| Total Fat **9g** | Unsaturated Fat **7g** | Sodium **168mg** | Dietary Fibre **5g** | Protein **5g** |

This **crisp and refreshing** salad showcases crunchy cucumber with a sweet-and-sour **honey vinegar dressing**.

Asian Cucumber Salad

 YIELD: **ABOUT 300G**   SERVING SIZE: **150G**   PREP TIME: **40 MINUTES**   COOK TIME: **0 MINUTES**

INGREDIENTS

2 medium cucumbers, sliced into (6mm) ¼-inch slices

1 tsp sea salt

40g (1½oz) red onion, thinly sliced

1 tbsp honey

1 tbsp white wine vinegar

1 tbsp sherry vinegar

METHOD

1 Put cucumber slices into a colander over a bowl or sink. Sprinkle with sea salt and let drain for 30 minutes.

2 Remove cucumber slices from the colander and squeeze out excess water with kitchen paper or a clean dish towel.

3 In a large bowl, combine cucumber and red onion.

4 In a small bowl, whisk together honey, white wine vinegar, and sherry vinegar.

5 Pour dressing over cucumber salad and toss to combine.

Storage: Cucumber salad is best enjoyed immediately.

Serving Suggestion: Serve cucumber salad as a side dish with Greek-Style Roast Chicken, Burgundy Lamb Kebabs, or Asian Turkey Lettuce Wraps.

Because cucumbers have a high water content, cucumber salads can often become soggy. Salting and draining the cucumbers removes excess water and allows them to absorb the tangy dressing.

NUTRITION

| Calories 84 | Saturated Fat 0g | Cholesterol 0mg | Carbohydrate 21g | Sugar 15g |
| Total Fat 0g | Unsaturated Fat 0g | Sodium 1,173mg | Dietary Fibre 2g | Protein 2g |

This **all-American garden salad** varies slightly from the traditional version, but still features many of the classic ingredients of this **lunchtime favourite**.

Grilled Chicken **Cobb Salad**

 YIELD: **ABOUT 1.8KG**   SERVING SIZE: **450G**   PREP TIME: **15 MINUTES**   COOK TIME: **10 MINUTES**

INGREDIENTS

- 3 x 170g (6oz) boneless, skinless chicken breasts
- 1 tbsp olive oil
- ¼ tsp sea salt
- 600g romaine lettuce, chopped
- 1 large avocado, chopped
- 15g (½ oz) parsley, chopped
- 6 slices bacon, cooked and chopped
- 300g (10½oz) cucumber, peeled and chopped
- 115g (4oz) spring onions, chopped

SPECIAL TOOLS

 GRILL OR GRILL PAN

METHOD

1 Place chicken breasts between two sheets of baking parchment. With a meat tenderizer, pound to an even thickness of 1.25cm (½ inch).

2 Brush both sides of chicken breasts with olive oil and season with sea salt.

3 Heat a grill to medium-high. Place chicken breasts on the grill and cook until browned on the bottom, about 3 to 5 minutes. Flip and cook until cooked through, about another 3 to 5 minutes.

4 Remove chicken from the grill and set aside to cool. When cool enough to touch, chop into bite-size pieces.

5 Place the romaine lettuce on each salad plate. Working in rows, top lettuce with avocado, parsley, bacon, cucumber, spring onions, and chicken.

Storage: Salad is best served immediately.

Serving Suggestion: Top with Greek Red Wine Vinaigrette.

For fast assembly, prep the chicken, bacon, and cucumber ahead of time and refrigerate until ready to use.

NUTRITION

Calories **325**	Saturated Fat **5g**	Cholesterol **53mg**	Carbohydrate **12g**	Sugar **3g**
Total Fat **20g**	Unsaturated Fat **10g**	Sodium **736mg**	Dietary Fibre **7g**	Protein **28g**

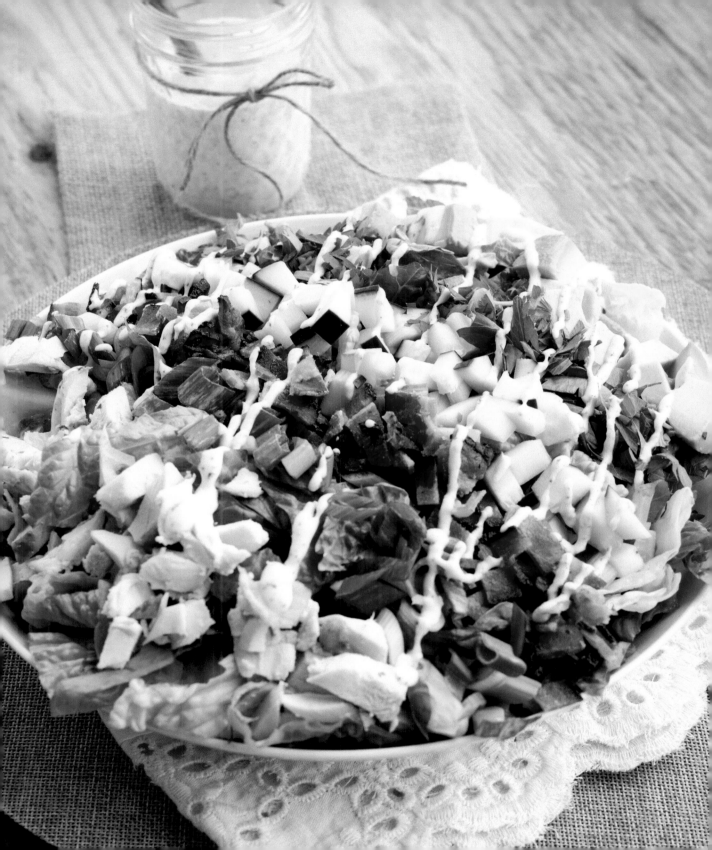

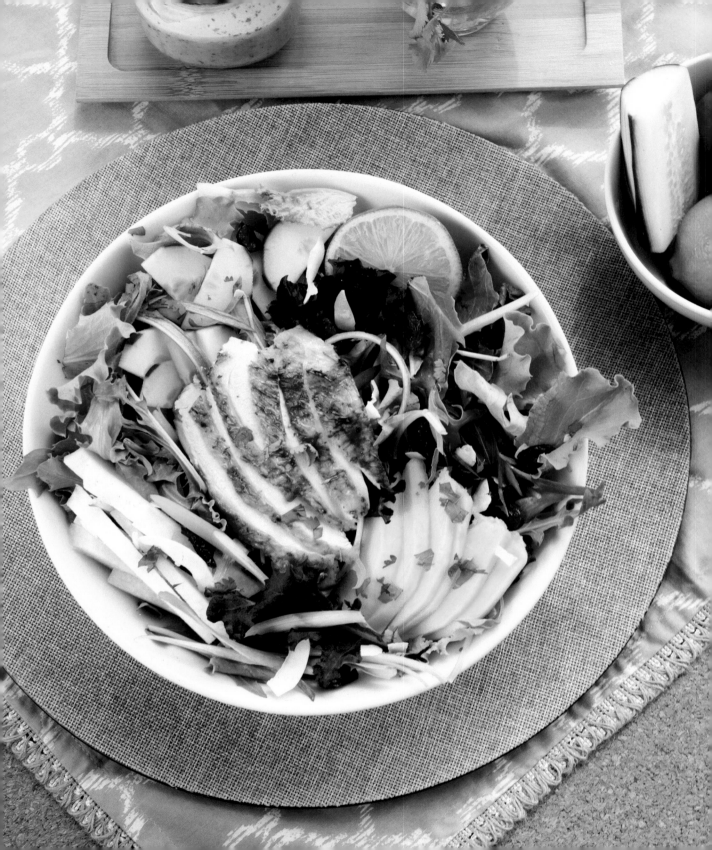

The **fresh tropical flavours** of mango and coconut pair perfectly with the refreshing texture of **jicama and cucumber** in this easy-to-assemble salad.

Caribbean Chicken Salad

 YIELD: **ABOUT 1.4KG**   SERVING SIZE: **350G**   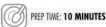 PREP TIME: **10 MINUTES**   COOK TIME: **10 MINUTES**

INGREDIENTS

- 3 x 170g (6oz) boneless, skinless chicken breasts
- 1 tbsp olive oil
- ¼ tsp sea salt
- 300g (10½oz) mixed greens
- 1 jicama (or crisp green apple), peeled and chopped
- 1 mango, peeled and sliced
- 1 cucumber, peeled and sliced
- 115g (4oz) spring onions, sliced
- 15g (½oz) unsweetened shredded coconut
- 30g (1oz) dried cranberries

SPECIAL TOOLS

 GRILL OR GRILL PAN

METHOD

1 Place chicken breasts between two sheets of baking parchment. With a meat tenderizer, pound to an even thickness of 1.25cm (½ inch).

2 Brush both sides of chicken breasts with olive oil and season with sea salt.

3 Heat grill to medium-high. Place chicken breasts under the grill and cook until browned on the bottom, about 3 to 5 minutes. Turn over and cook until cooked through, about 3 to 5 minutes more.

4 Remove chicken from grill and let cool. When cool enough to touch, slice into strips.

5 In a large bowl, toss mixed greens, jicama, mango, cucumber, and spring onions to combine.

6 Top salad with sliced chicken, shredded coconut, and cranberries.

Storage: Salad is best served immediately.

Serving Suggestion: Serve salad with Coriander Lime Vinaigrette or Sweet Red Raspberry Vinaigrette.

Jicama is a bulbous tuber with crisp, white flesh. It tastes like a cross between a sweet pear and a starchy potato. Peeled and chopped, it can be used raw or cooked in soups and stir-fries.

NUTRITION

Calories **303**
Total Fat **8g**
Saturated Fat **3g**
Unsaturated Fat **4g**
Cholesterol **45g**
Sodium **539mg**
Carbohydrate **36g**
Dietary Fibre **12g**
Sugar **17g**
Protein **25g**

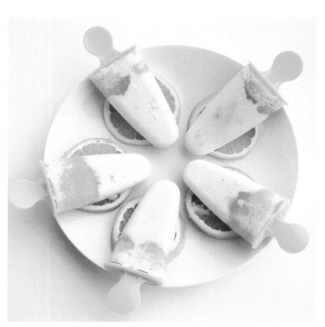
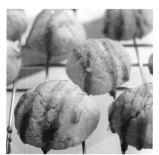
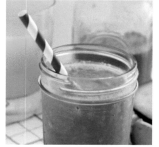

CHAPTER 8
Desserts
& Beverages

Enjoy the **buttery** flavours of **caramel** without the heavy cream. This **decadent, salt-kissed sauce** is the perfect accompaniment to any dessert.

Sea Salt **Caramel Sauce**

 YIELD: **175ML**   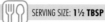 SERVING SIZE: **1½ TBSP**   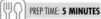 PREP TIME: **5 MINUTES**   COOK TIME: **10 MINUTES**

INGREDIENTS

50ml (2fl oz) cup coconut cream

50ml (2fl oz) honey

2 tbsp coconut sugar

1 tbsp vanilla extract

Dash sea salt

1 tbsp ghee

METHOD

1 In a small saucepan over medium heat, bring coconut cream, honey, and coconut sugar to the boil.

2 Add vanilla extract and sea salt and reduce heat to low.

3 Simmer for 5 minutes, stirring frequently.

4 Remove from heat and stir in ghee until melted and combined.

Storage: Enjoy warm immediately, or refrigerate for up to 1 month.

Serving Suggestion: Drizzle Sea Salt Caramel Coconut Sauce over fresh fruit, serve as a dip with Cinnamon Apple Crisps, or use to make Caramel Coconut Macaroons.

To make your own coconut cream, refrigerate a can of full-fat coconut milk overnight. The thick cream will rise to the top; you can then separate it from the remaining liquid portion.

NUTRITION

Calories 78	Saturated Fat 2g	Cholesterol 4mg	Carbohydrate 12g	Sugar 12g
Total Fat 3g	Unsaturated Fat 10g	Sodium 22mg	Dietary Fibre 0g	Protein 0g

When whipped with a little sweetener, **coconut cream is transformed** into a **light, fluffy,** and **delicious** dessert topping.

Coconut Whipped Cream

 YIELD: **350ML**   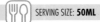 SERVING SIZE: **50ML**   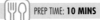 PREP TIME: **10 MINS**   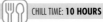 CHILL TIME: **10 HOURS**

INGREDIENTS

1 x 400ml can full-fat coconut milk

50ml (2fl oz) coconut water

3 tbsp maple syrup

SPECIAL TOOLS

 MIXER

METHOD

1 Place the can of full-fat coconut milk in the fridge and chill overnight.

2 Chill a metal mixing bowl in the freezer for 5 minutes.

3 Scoop coconut cream out of can and into the chilled bowl, leaving behind coconut water that has settled to the bottom of the can.

4 Whip coconut cream with electric mixer on low until creamy (about 1 minute).

5 Add coconut water and maple syrup and continue whipping until light and fluffy (about 2 minutes).

Storage: Store in the refrigerator for up to 3 days.

Serving Suggestion: Serve on top of fresh berries.

NUTRITION

| Calories 146 | Saturated Fat 10g | Cholesterol 0mg | Carbohydrate 9g | Sugar 8g |
| Total Fat 12g | Unsaturated Fat 0g | Sodium 16mg | Dietary Fibre 0g | Protein 0g |

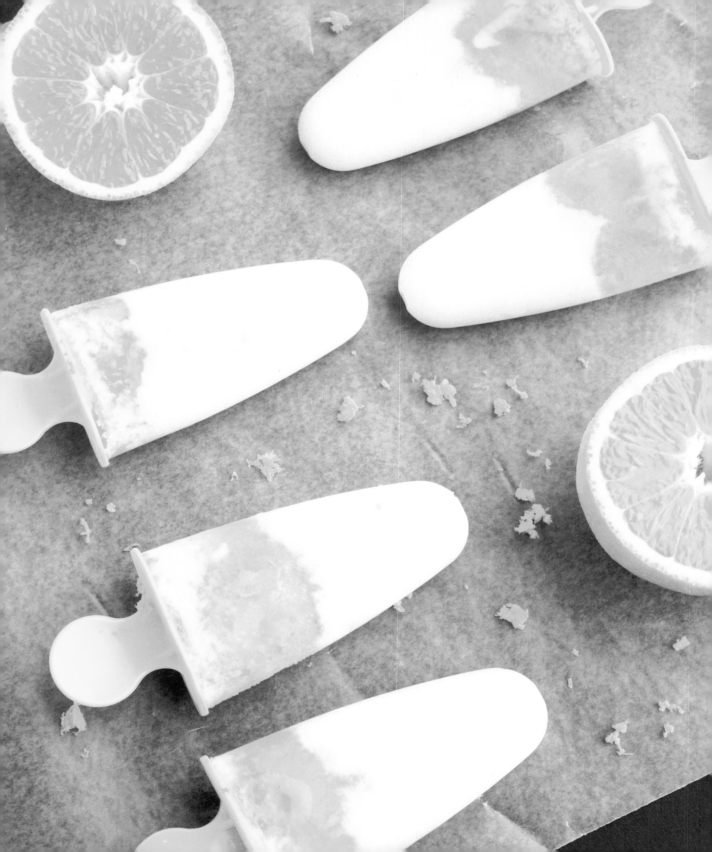

This **dairy-free frozen fruit lolly** combines creamy coconut milk and freshly squeezed orange juice for an AIP twist on the **classic summer favourite.**

Orange **Cream Ice Lolly**

 YIELD: **12 LOLLIES**   SERVING SIZE: **1 LOLLY**   PREP TIME: **20 MINUTES**   CHILL TIME: **12–24 HOURS**

INGREDIENTS

1 x 400ml can light coconut milk

4 tbsp maple syrup

225ml (8fl oz) freshly squeezed orange juice

1 tbsp orange zest

SPECIAL TOOLS

 ICE LOLLY MOULDS

METHOD

1 In a large bowl, whisk together coconut milk and 2 tablespoons maple syrup until smooth.

2 Pour coconut mixture into ice lolly mould, filling each mould halfway. Freeze for 10 minutes.

3 In a small bowl, whisk together orange juice, orange zest, and remaining 2 tablespoons maple syrup.

4 Remove coconut mixture from the freezer, pour orange juice mixture into the moulds, and insert the sticks. Freeze for 12 to 24 hours or until frozen through.

Storage: Store in the freezer for up to 3 months.

Variation: To make Strawberry Banana Fruit Lollies, replace orange juice mixture with 225g (8oz) strawberry purée and 50g (1¾oz) chopped banana.

Don't have an ice lolly mould? Use plastic cups and wooden treat sticks instead.

NUTRITION

| Calories 47 | Saturated Fat 2g | Cholesterol 0mg | Carbohydrate 7g | Sugar 7g |
| Total Fat 2g | Unsaturated Fat 0g | Sodium 1mg | Dietary Fibre 0g | Protein 0g |

This **cosy dessert** is a healthy alternative to baked apple pie and features all of the same **sweet and spicy autumn flavours**.

Warm Cinnamon Apples

 YIELD: **260G**   SERVING SIZE: **65G**   PREP TIME: **2 MINUTES**   COOK TIME: **20 MINUTES**

INGREDIENTS

1 tbsp ghee

2 medium apples, peeled and chopped

75g (3oz) raisins

2 tbsp maple syrup

1 tsp vanilla extract

¼ tsp cinnamon

METHOD

1 In a large frying pan, heat ghee over a medium heat.

2 Add apples, raisins, maple syrup, vanilla extract, and cinnamon. Stir to combine.

3 Cover and cook for 20 minutes or until apples are fork-tender.

Storage: Store in the fridge for up to 3 days.

Serving Suggestion: Serve with Coconut Whipped Cream for a warm, satisfying dessert.

NUTRITION

Calories 168	Saturated Fat 2g	Cholesterol 8mg	Carbohydrate 36g	Sugar 29g
Total Fat 4g	Unsaturated Fat 1g	Sodium 4mg	Dietary Fibre 3g	Protein 1g

Frying bananas in coconut oil gives them a **crisp and caramelized** exterior with a **warm and creamy centre**.

Honey Fried Bananas

 YIELD: **2 BANANAS**   SERVING SIZE: ½ **BANANA** 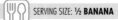 PREP TIME: **2 MINUTES**   COOK TIME: **5 MINUTES**

INGREDIENTS

- 125ml (4fl oz) warm water
- 1 tbsp honey
- 2 tbsp coconut oil
- 2 medium underripe bananas, peeled and sliced
- ⅛ tsp cinnamon

METHOD

1 In a small bowl, whisk together warm water and honey.

2 Heat coconut oil in a large frying pan over a medium-high heat.

3 Add banana slices and fry for 2 minutes. Flip and fry for another 2 minutes or until bananas are a crisp golden brown on both sides.

4 Remove the pan from heat and pour honey-water mixture over bananas.

5 Sprinkle with cinnamon and let cool slightly before serving.

Storage: Fried bananas are best served immediately.

Serving Suggestion: Serve with Coconut Whipped Cream or atop Pumpkin Spice Ice Cream.

NUTRITION

Calories **127**	Saturated Fat **6g**	Cholesterol **0mg**	Carbohydrate **18g**	Sugar **12g**
Total Fat **7g**	Unsaturated Fat **0g**	Sodium **1mg**	Dietary Fibre **2g**	Protein **1g**

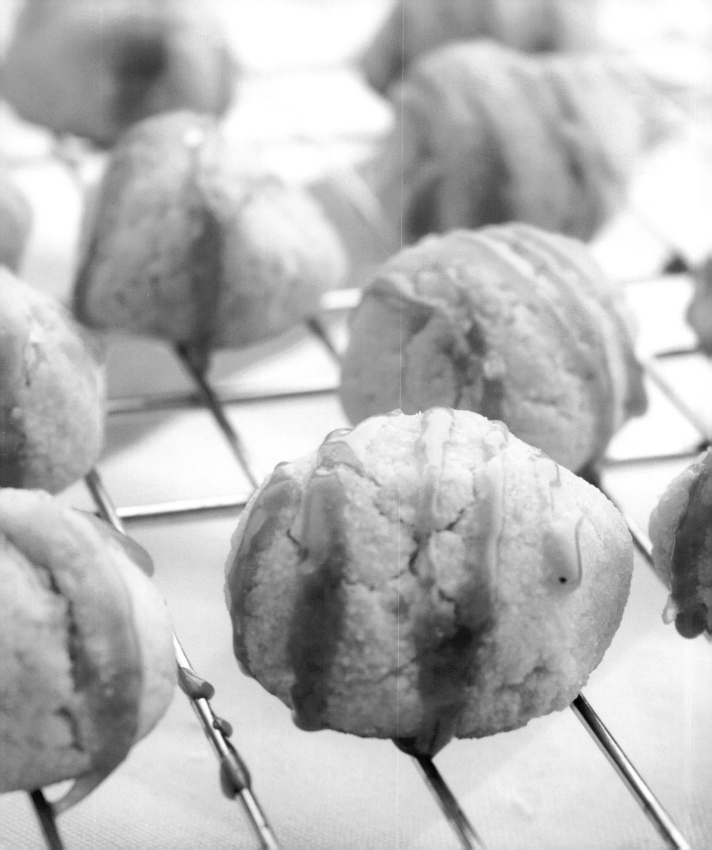

These **chewy, bite-size treats** combine the sweetness of coconut and maple syrup with sea salt for a mouthful of flavour.

Caramel Coconut
Macaroons

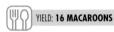 YIELD: **16 MACAROONS**   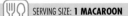 SERVING SIZE: **1 MACAROON**   PREP TIME: **5 MINUTES**   COOK TIME: **15 MINUTES**

INGREDIENTS

90g (3¼oz) unsweetened shredded coconut

2 tbsp coconut oil

2 tbsp coconut flour

1 tbsp vanilla extract

50ml (2fl oz) maple syrup

¼ tsp sea salt

50ml (2fl oz) **Sea Salt Caramel Sauce**

SPECIAL TOOLS

 FOOD PROCESSOR

METHOD

1 Preheat the oven to 180°C (350°F/Gas 4). Line a baking tray with baking parchment.

2 In a food processor, combine shredded coconut, coconut oil, coconut flour, vanilla extract, maple syrup, and sea salt. Process for 30 seconds or until ingredients are well combined and have the texture of wet sand.

3 Scoop batter onto the baking tray in 1-tablespoon portions.

4 Bake for 10 minutes. Rotate the pan and bake for another 5 minutes or until golden brown.

5 Let cool on pan for 5 to 10 minutes before transferring to wire rack. When completely cool, drizzle with Sea Salt Caramel Sauce.

Storage: Store in an airtight container for up to 1 week.

NUTRITION

Calories 59	Saturated Fat 4g	Cholesterol 0mg	Carbohydrate 5g	Sugar 4g
Total Fat 4g	Unsaturated Fat 0g	Sodium 39mg	Dietary Fibre 1g	Protein 1g

Get your greens easily with this nutrient-packed beverage. Avocado adds the perfect creamy texture to this **citrusy green smoothie**.

Avocado Pineapple
Smoothie

 YIELD: **300ML**   SERVING SIZE: **300ML**   PREP TIME: **2 MINUTES**   COOK TIME: **NONE**

INGREDIENTS

75g (2¾oz) kale, chopped and tightly packed

225ml (8fl oz) orange juice

115g (4oz) pineapple, roughly chopped

50g (1¾oz) avocado, chopped

4–5 ice cubes

METHOD

1 In a blender, combine kale, orange juice, pineapple, avocado, and ice cubes.

2 Blend for 30 seconds or until smooth.

Storage: Smoothies are best enjoyed immediately.

SPECIAL TOOLS

 BLENDER

NUTRITION

| Calories 218 | Saturated Fat 1g | Cholesterol 0mg | Carbohydrate 34g | Sugar 18g |
| Total Fat 9g | Unsaturated Fat 10g | Sodium 34mg | Dietary Fibre 6g | Protein 5g |

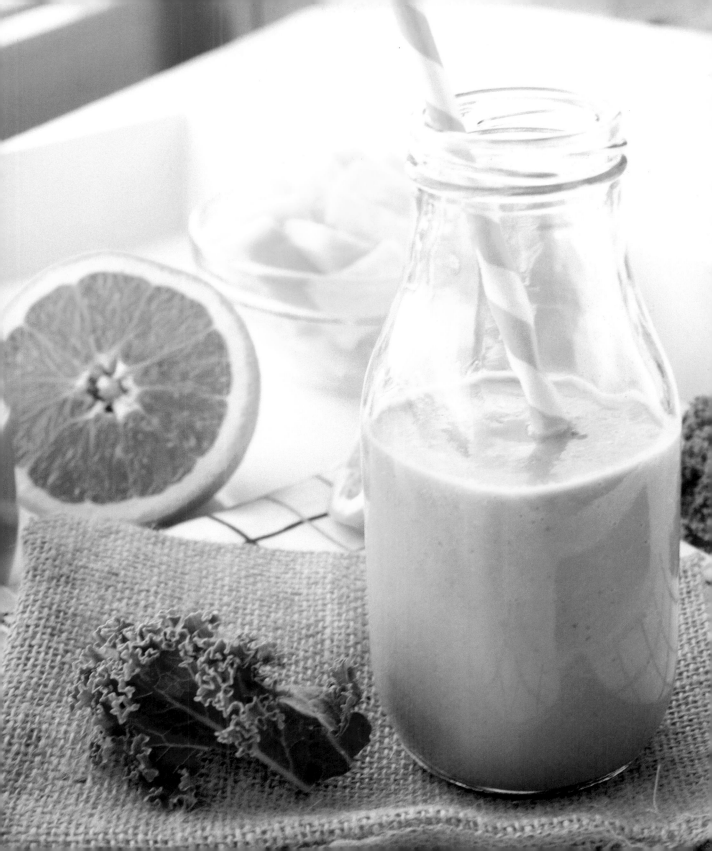

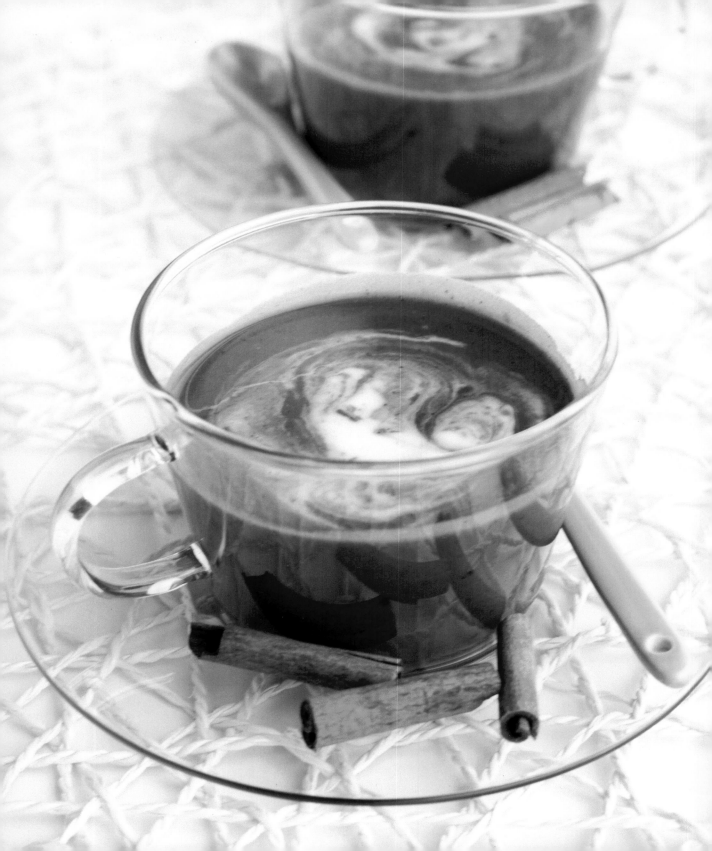

Enjoy a warm cup of hot "cocoa" on a cold day with this **dairy-free coconut milk** version featuring **rich carob powder** and **sweet maple syrup**.

Creamy Coconut Milk
Hot Cocoa

 YIELD: **450ML**    SERVING SIZE: **225ml**   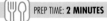 PREP TIME: **2 MINUTES**   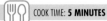 COOK TIME: **5 MINUTES**

INGREDIENTS

450ml (16fl oz) light coconut milk

2 tbsp carob powder

2 tbsp maple syrup

1 tsp vanilla extract

½ tsp cinnamon

50ml (2fl oz) water

METHOD

1 In a small saucepan over a low heat, whisk together coconut milk, carob powder, maple syrup, vanilla extract, cinnamon, and water.

2 Heat for 5 minutes, stirring frequently, until contents are combined and warm.

Storage: Cocoa is best served immediately.

Serving Suggestion: Serve warm topped with a dollop of Coconut Whipped Cream.

NUTRITION

Calories 241	Saturated Fat 11g	Cholesterol 0mg	Carbohydrate 39g	Sugar 27g
Total Fat 12g	Unsaturated Fat 0g	Sodium 82mg	Dietary Fibre 9g	Protein 1g

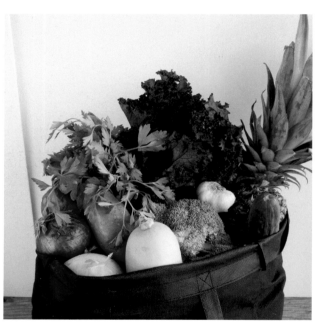
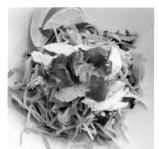
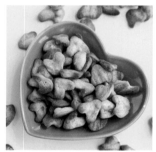

CHAPTER 9

Meal Plans

& Shopping Lists

Using Meal Plans
and Shopping Lists

The following pages include six weeks of meal plans, along with shopping lists, to guide you in considering what to eat during the weeks ahead.

About the Meals

Whether you are new to the AIP diet or are looking for some new recipes to spice up your meals, the meal plans for each week are structured to maximize your time and leftovers while still offering variety.

Breakfasts
Each week includes two different breakfast options. Breakfast items can all be made ahead of time.

Lunches
Lunches are either simple salads that can be prepped ahead of time or meals from a previous night's dinner.

Dinners
More complex dinner recipes are scheduled for the weekend, while easier recipes are suggested for weeknight meals.

About the Shopping Lists

Each plan is accompanied by a corresponding shopping list to make your life easier.

Quantities: Each shopping list includes the exact quantities of ingredients needed for all of the recipes within the week.

Inventory: Before you go shopping, take an inventory of your current fridge, freezer, and store cupboard and cross off items you already have to avoid overbuying.

Staples: Many of the weekly meal plans include staple recipes like Worcestershire Sauce and Seed-Free Curry Powder. If you already have these on hand, eliminate those ingredients from the shopping list.

Avoid Temptation

Avoid the temptation of foods that are not AIP-friendly by visiting the supermarket less frequently.
Try shopping only once a week, and choose a day when you have time to peruse the shelves consciously and carefully.

Things to **Consider**

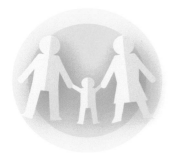

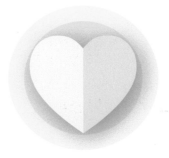

Family Size Depending on how many individuals you cook for in your household, some of these recipes may stretch further than what's listed. Take this opportunity to freeze leftovers for when you need a meal in a pinch.

New Recipes vs. Leftovers The meal plans are structured to make the most of leftovers. Note that recipes in **bold** need to be made from scratch.

Perfect Pairings Many main course recipes are paired with side dish recipes to create a complete meal. These side dishes are simply suggestions, so feel free to mix and match different side dishes to the main courses as you begin to identify your favourite recipes.

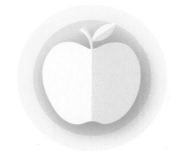

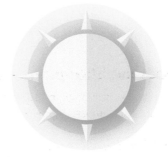

Tools and Appliances Each recipe lists any special tools needed to create the dish. Reference each recipe to ensure you have the necessary tools to make a dish before you begin your planning and shopping.

Fruit and Salads If you require larger serving sizes than those suggested throughout the book, feel free to double the serving size, or add something simple to the meal, such as fresh fruit to your breakfast or a side salad with your dinner.

Practice and Have Fun! The more you practice, the easier planning becomes. The AIP diet is an opportunity for you to try new foods, build a list of your favourite go-to recipes, and involve your friends and family in your new way of cooking and eating.

Week 1 Meal Plan

	SUNDAY	**MONDAY**	**TUESDAY**
BREAKFAST	Crisp Ham Cups; Root Vegetable Breakfast Hash	Key Lime No'gurt	Crisp Ham Cups; Root Vegetable Breakfast Hash
LUNCH	Mediterranean Tuna Salad	Wild Mushroom and Meatball Stew	Mediterranean Tuna Salad
DINNER	Wild Mushroom and Meatball Stew	Herbed Baked Spaghetti; Squash; Tomato-Less Pasta Sauce	Middle Eastern Bison Burgers; Sea Salt Kale Crisps

Shopping List

Proteins
- Deli ham (12 slices)
- Pancetta (55g; 2oz)
- Minced pork (450g; 1lb)
- Minced bison (450g; 1lb)
- Minced turkey, dark meat (450g; 1lb)
- Salmon fillet, skin on (450g; 1lb)

Produce
- Onions (4)
- Red onion (1)
- Shallot (1)
- Garlic (17 cloves)
- Spring onions (6)
- Parsley (25g; 1oz)
- Fresh thyme (5g)
- Chives (½ tbsp)
- Fresh rosemary (3 tbsp)
- Fresh oregano (1 tbsp)
- Fresh ginger (2 tbsp)
- Fresh basil (5g)
- Sweet potato (1)
- Swede (1)

- Carrots (5)
- Parsnip (1)
- Beetroot (1 small)
- Spaghetti squash (1 medium)
- Avocados (3)
- Cucumber (½)
- Cauliflower (1 head)
- Celery (2 stalks)
- Lime (1)
- Lemon (1)
- Mushrooms (800g; 1lb 12oz)
- Kale (800g; 1lb 12oz)

- Fennel (½ bulb)
- Butterhead lettuce (2 heads; about 16 large leaves)
- Pineapple (450g; 1lb))

WEDNESDAY	THURSDAY	FRIDAY	SATURDAY
Key Lime No'gurt	Crisp Ham Cups; Root Vegetable Breakfast Hash	Key Lime No'gurt	Crisp Ham Cups; Root Vegetable Breakfast Hash
Middle Eastern Bison Burgers; Sea Salt Kale Crisps	Mediterranean Tuna Salad	Wild Mushroom and Meatball Stew	Pineapple Teriyaki Salmon; Cauliflower Fried Rice
Herbed Baked Spaghetti; Squash; Tomato-Less Pasta Sauce	**Asian Turkey Lettuce Wraps**	**Pineapple Teriyaki Salmon; Cauliflower Fried Rice**	Asian Turkey Lettuce Wraps

Store Cupboard

- Olive oil (225ml; 8fl oz)
- Coconut oil (1 tbsp)
- Ghee (4 tbsp)
- Cider vinegar (225ml; 8fl oz)
- Balsamic vinegar (1 tbsp)
- Coconut aminos (¾ cup)
- Fish sauce (3 tbsp)
- Maple syrup (125ml; 4fl oz)
- Honey (3 tbsp)
- Molasses (1 tbsp)
- Lime juice (3 tbsp)
- Lemon juice (50ml; 2fl oz)
- Beef stock (900ml; 1½ pints)
- Vegetable stock (450ml; 16fl oz)
- Sweet potato purée (2 tbsp)
- Water chestnuts (1 x 113g can)
- Arrowroot powder (2 tbsp)
- Albacore tuna (4 x170g cans)
- Artichoke hearts (1 x 395g can)
- Green olives (¾ cup)
- Worcestershire Sauce

Spices and Others

- Sea salt (3⅛ tbsp)
- Dried basil (2 tbsp)
- Dried thyme (1 tbsp)
- Dried oregano (2 tbsp)
- Onion powder (2 tbsp)
- Garlic powder (1¾ tbsp)
- Dried turmeric (1½ tbsp)
- Dried coriander (1 tbsp)
- Dried dill (½ tbsp)
- Ground cinnamon (½ tbsp)
- Ground ginger (½ tbsp)
- Ground cloves (¾ tbsp)
- Seed-Free Curry Powder
- Pitted prunes (about 10)
- Bacon fat (2 tbsp)

Week 2 Meal Plan

	SUNDAY	MONDAY	TUESDAY
BREAKFAST	Apple Cinnamon Hearts Cereal	Rosemary and Thyme Sausage Patties; Root Vegetable Breakfast Hash	Apple Cinnamon Hearts Cereal
LUNCH	Avocado Chicken Salad	Triple-Berry Barbecue Ribs; Honey Vinegar Tri-Coloured Slaw	Roasted Butternut Squash and Sage Soup; Celeriac Apple Currant Slaw
DINNER	Triple-Berry Barbecue Ribs; Honey Vinegar Tri-Coloured Slaw	Roasted Butternut Squash and Sage Soup; Celeriac Apple Currant Slaw	Greek-Style Roast Chicken

Shopping List

Proteins
- Minced pork (450g; 1lb)
- Lamb stewing meat (2 lb; 450g)
- Whole roasting chicken, without giblets (2.1kg; 4½lb)
- Rack ribs (1.5kg; 3lb)
- Boneless, skinless, chicken breast (450g; 1lb)

Produce
- Yellow onions (3)
- Red onions (2)
- Spring onions (6)
- Shallots (2)
- Garlic (23 cloves)
- Fresh rosemary (2 tsp)
- Fresh thyme (1 tbsp + 2 tsp)
- Fresh sage (7g)
- Chives (½ tsp)
- Fresh basil (2 tbsp)
- Fresh coriander (35g; 1¼oz)
- Fresh ginger (1 tsp)

- Sweet potatoes (3 medium)
- Celeriac (4 cups)
- Swede (1)
- Carrots (5)
- Parsnip (1)
- Granny Smith or similar apples (3)
- Butternut squash (1 medium)
- Limes (1½)
- Lemons (5)
- Mixed greens (300g; 10½oz)

- Cucumbers (3½)
- Jicama (1)
- Red cabbage (300g; 10½oz)
- Green cabbage (300g; 10½oz)
- Avocados (2)
- Mango (1)
- Strawberries (70g; 2½oz)
- Blueberries (35g; 1¼oz)
- Cherries, frozen (70g; 2½oz)

WEDNESDAY	THURSDAY	FRIDAY	SATURDAY
Rosemary and Thyme Sausage Patties; Root Vegetable Breakfast Hash	Apple Cinnamon Hearts Cereal	Rosemary and Thyme Sausage Patties; Root Vegetable Breakfast Hash	Apple Cinnamon Hearts Cereal
Caribbean Chicken Salad; Coriander Lime Vinagrette	Avacado Chicken Salad	Roasted Butternut Squash and Sage Soup; Celeriac Apple Currant Slaw	Burgundy Lamb Kebabs; Asian Cucumber Salad
Burgundy Lamb Kebabs; Asian Cucumber Salad	Greek-Style Roast Chicken	Burgundy Lamb Kebabs; Asian Cucumber Salad	Caribbean Chicken Salad; Coriander Lime Vinagrette

Store Cupboard

- Olive oil (300ml; 10fl oz)
- Coconut oil (50ml; 2fl oz)
- Ghee (2 tbsp)
- White wine vinegar (1 tbsp)
- Sherry vinegar (1 tbsp)
- Apple cider vinegar (175ml; 6fl oz)
- Coconut aminos (2 tbsp)
- Fish sauce (2 tbsp)
- Honey (80ml; 3fl oz)
- Maple syrup (140ml; 4½fl oz)
- Molasses (3 tbsp)
- Lime juice (50ml; 2fl oz)
- Bone Broth or chicken stock (1 litre; 1¾ pints)
- Beef stock (225ml; 8fl oz)
- Light coconut milk (225ml; 8fl oz)
- Coconut flour (60g; 2¼oz)
- Arrowroot powder (65g; 2½oz)
- Triple-Berry Barbecue Sauce
- Worcestershire Sauce

Spices and Others

- Sea salt (5½ tsp)
- Ground cinnamon (1 tsp)
- Dried parsley (1½ tbsp)
- Dried oregano (2 tbsp)
- Garlic powder (½ tsp)
- Onion powder (¾ tsp)
- Ground cloves (¼ tsp)
- Vanilla extract (2 tsp)

- Bacon fat (3 tbsp)
- Unsweetened applesauce (250g; 9oz)
- Orange juice (50ml; 2 fl oz)

- Currants (75g; 2¾oz)
- Dried cranberries (30g; 1oz)
- Unsweetened shredded coconut (15g; ½oz)
- Red wine (225ml; 8fl oz)

Week 3 Meal Plan

	SUNDAY	MONDAY	TUESDAY
BREAKFAST	Carrot Cake Waffles	Sweet & Spicy Gra'no'la	Carrot Cake Waffles
LUNCH	Tuscan Sausage and Kale Soup; Hasselback Sweet Potatoes	Grilled Chicken Cobb Salad; Greek Red Wine Vinaigrette	Tuscan Sausage and Kale Soup; Hasselback Sweet Potatoes
DINNER	Blackened Chicken Breast; Pad Thai Noodles	Chimichurri Skirt Steak; Hasselback Sweet Potatoes	Orange Pulled Pork Carnitas; Pan-Seared Brussels Sprouts with Bacon

Shopping List

Proteins

- Skirt steak (450g; 1lb)
- Pork sausage (225g; ½lb)
- Bacon (10 slices)
- Boneless pork shoulder (1.6kg; 3½lb)
- Boneless pork tenderloin (450g; 1lb)
- Boneless, skinless chicken breast (900g; 2lb)

Produce

- Yellow onion (1)
- White onion (1)
- Red onion (1)
- Shallot (½)
- Spring onions (6)
- Garlic (21 cloves)
- Fresh rosemary (1 tbsp)
- Fresh sage (1 tbsp)
- Parsley (65g; 2½oz)
- Fresh coriander (15g; ½oz)

- Sweet potatoes (4 medium)
- Carrots (900g; 2lb)
- Butternut squash (200g;7oz)
- Plantains, ripe or green (600g; 1lb 5oz)
- Avocado (1)
- Cucumber (300g; 10½ oz)
- Courgette (1)
- Brussels sprouts (450g;1lb)

- Kale (140g; 5oz)
- Broccoli (255g; 9oz)
- Romaine lettuce (400g; 14oz)
- Rocket (50g; 2 oz)
- Lime (1)
- Orange (1)

WEDNESDAY	THURSDAY	FRIDAY	SATURDAY
Sweet & Spicy Gra'no'la	Carrot Cake Waffles	Sweet & Spicy Gra'no'la	Carrot Cake Waffles
Blackened Chicken Breast; Pad Thai Noodles	Grilled Chicken Cobb Salad; Greek Red Wine Vinaigrette	Pork Tenderloin with Roasted Carrot Romesco	Tuscan Sausage and Kale Soup; Hasselback Sweet Potatoes
Chimichurri Skirt Steak; Hasselback Sweet Potatoes	**Pork Tenderloin with Roasted Carrot Romesco**	Orange Pulled Pork Carnitas; Pan-Seared Brussels Sprouts with Bacon	Orange Pulled Pork Carnitas; Pan-Seared Brussels Sprouts with Bacon

Store Cupboard

- Olive oil (255ml; 9fl oz)
- Coconut oil (95ml; 3fl oz)
- Ghee (3 tbsp)
- Cider vinegar (2 tbsp)
- Red wine vinegar (50ml; 2fl oz)
- Sherry vinegar (3 tbsp)
- Lime juice (50ml; 2fl oz)
- Lemon juice (65ml; 2¼fl oz)
- Coconut aminos (2 tbsp)
- Fish sauce (50ml; 2 fl oz)

- Maple syrup (50ml; 2fl oz)
- Coconut butter (1 tbsp)
- Chicken stock (900ml; 1½ pints)
- Light coconut milk (125ml; 4fl oz)
- Pumpkin purée (½ cup)
- Sweet potato purée (125g; 4½oz)
- Arrowroot powder (65g; 2½oz)
- Bicarbonate of soda (2 tsp)

Spices and Others

- Sea salt (3 tsp)
- Cinnamon (2 tsp)
- Cream of tartar (1 tsp)
- Ground ginger (1 tsp)
- Bay leaves (2)
- Dried oregano (4 tbsp + ½ tsp)
- Dried thyme (1½ tsp)
- Garlic powder (3 tsp)
- Onion powder (1½ tsp)
- Dried turmeric (1½ tsp)
- Dried coriander (1 tsp)
- Dried basil (1 tsp)
- Dried dill (½ tsp)

- Ground cloves (¼ tsp)
- Seed-Free Curry Powder

- Unsweetened banana chips (55g; 2½oz)
- Unsweetened dried mango (55g; 2½oz)
- Raisins (75g; 2¾oz)
- Unsweetened coconut flakes (150g; 5½oz)
- Coconut sugar (1½ tsp)

Week 4 Meal Plan

	SUNDAY	MONDAY	TUESDAY
BREAKFAST	Okonomiyaki	Zesty Lemon No'gurt	Okonomiyaki
LUNCH	Wild Mushroom Sausage Stew	Sunday Slow Cooker Pot Roast; Parsnip Purée	Meatloaf Muffins; Cranberry Orange Relish
DINNER	Sunday Slow Cooker Pot Roast; Parsnip Purée	Meatloaf Muffins; Cranberry Orange Relish	Apple Glazed Pork Chops; Roasted Balsamic Green Beans

Shopping List

Proteins

- Bacon (6 slices)
- Bone-in pork chops (450g; 1lb)
- Skirt steak (450g; 1lb)
- Boneless braising steak (1.5kg; 3lb)
- Minced beef (450g; 1lb)
- Pork sausages (4)

Produce

- Yellow onions (4)
- Shallots (300g; 10½oz)
- Garlic (23 cloves)
- Spring onions (6)
- Leeks (2)
- Fresh thyme (3 tbsp + 1 tsp)
- Fresh ginger (1 tbsp + 1 tsp)
- Parsley (25g; 1 oz)
- Carrots (2 medium)
- Mint (1 tbsp)
- Sweet potatoes (3 large)
- Parsnips (8)

- Celery (3 stalks)
- Courgette (1)
- Green cabbage (300g; 10½oz)
- Cauliflower (2 medium heads)
- Broccoli (1 small head)
- Green beans (450g; 1lb)
- Avocados (2)
- Apples (2 large)
- Oranges (2)
- Grapefruit (1)

- Pomegranate (1)
- Lemon (1)
- Whole cranberries (480g; 1lb 1oz)
- Mushrooms (300g; 10½oz)

WEDNESDAY	THURSDAY	FRIDAY	SATURDAY
Zesty Lemon No'gurt	Okonomiyaki	Zesty Lemon No'gurt	Okonomiyaki
Sunday Slow Cooker Pot Roast; Parsnip Purée	Broccoli Beef Stir-Fry; Cauliflower Fried Rice	Wild Mushroom Sausage Stew	Cauliflower Leek Soup; Citrus Mint Salad
Broccoli Beef Stir-Fry, Cauliflower Fried Rice	Apple Glazed Pork Chops; Roasted Balsamic Green Beans	**Cauliflower Leek Soup; Citrus Mint Salad**	Parsnip Seafood Chowder

Pantry Items

- Olive oil (100ml; 4 fl oz)
- Coconut oil (2 tbsp)
- Ghee (150ml; 6fl oz)
- Balsamic vinegar (4 tsp)
- White wine vinegar (1 tsp)
- Cider vinegar (140ml; 5fl oz)
- Coconut aminos (140ml; 5fl oz)
- Fish sauce (50ml; 2fl oz)
- Lemon juice (3 tbsp + 1 tsp)
- Lime juice (3 tbsp)
- Maple syrup (355ml; 12fl oz)
- Honey (50ml; 2fl oz)
- Molasses (1 tbsp)
- Chicken stock (1.1 litres; 2 pints)
- Vegetable stock (100ml; 4 fl oz)
- Beef broth (450ml;16 fl oz)
- Apple sauce (85g; 3oz)
- Light coconut milk (2½ x 400ml cans)
- Coconut flour (55g; 2oz)
- Arrowroot powder (1 tsp)
- Tapioca starch (20g; ¾oz)
- Worcestershire Sauce
- Beef stock (900ml; 1½ pints)

Spices and Others

- Sea salt (3 tsp)
- Cinnamon (2 tsp)
- Cream of tartar (1 tsp)
- Ground ginger (1 tsp)
- Bay leaf (1)
- Dried oregano (4 tbsp + ½ tsp)
- Dried thyme (1½ tsp)
- Garlic powder (3 tsp)
- Onion powder (1½ tsp)
- Dried turmeric (1½ tsp)
- Dried coriander (1 tsp)
- Dried basil (1 tsp)
- Dried dill (½ tsp)
- Ground cloves (¼ tsp)
- Parsley (15; ½ oz)

- Unsweetened banana chips (55g; 2oz)
- Unsweetened dried mango (55g; 2oz)
- Sultanas (75g; 2¾oz)
- Unsweetened coconut flakes (150g; 5½oz)
- Coconut sugar (1½ tsp)

Week 5 Meal Plan

	SUNDAY	MONDAY	TUESDAY
BREAKFAST	Apple Cinnamon No-Oat Oatmeal	Carrot Cake Waffles	Apple Cinnamon No-Oat Oatmeal
LUNCH	Shaved Broccoli and Cauliflower Slaw	Bacon-Wrapped Scallops; Roasted Tenderstem with White Wine Mushrooms	Crispy Chicken Strips with Mango Honey Sauce; Rosemary Sweet Potato Crisps
DINNER	Bacon-Wrapped Scallops; Roasted Tenderstem with White Wine Mushrooms	Crispy Chicken Strips with Mango Honey Sauce; Rosemary Sweet Potato Chips	Honey Ginger Glazed Salmon; Swede Purée

Shopping List

Proteins

- Large sea scallops (450g; 1lb)
- Bacon (12 slices)
- Pancetta (55g; 2oz)
- Boneless, skinless chicken breast (450g; 1lb)
- Salmon fillet, skin on (450g; 1lb)

Produce

- Shallot (1 medium)
- Spring onions (5)
- Garlic (7 cloves)
- Fresh coriander (2 tbsp)
- Fresh basil (30g; 1oz)
- Fresh ginger (1 tbsp)
- Parsley (25g; 1oz)
- Fresh rosemary (2 tbsp)
- Sweet potatoes (2 medium)
- Swede (1)
- Butternut squash (½)
- Carrots (6)
- Broccoli (1 large head)

- Tenderstem broccoli (2 bunches)
- Cauliflower (2 heads)
- Courgette (8 medium)
- Baby bella mushrooms (225g; 8oz)
- Kale (1 large bunch)
- Avocado (1)
- Plantains (2)
- Lime (1)
- Lemon (1)
- Orange (1)
- Mango (1)

WEDNESDAY	THURSDAY	FRIDAY	SATURDAY
Carrot Cake Waffles	Apple Cinnamon No-Oat Oatmeal	Carrot Cake Waffles	Apple Cinnamon No-Oat Oatmeal
Shaved Broccoli and Cauliflower Slaw	**Classic Kale Salad**	Classic Kale Salad	Crispy Chicken Strips with Mango Honey Sauce; Rosemary Sweet Potato Crisps
Honey Ginger Glazed Salmon; Swede Purée	**Garlic Pesto Courgette Pasta**	Garlic Pesto Courgette Pasta	Shaved Broccoli and Cauliflower Slaw

Store Cupboard 1

- Olive oil (415ml; 14½fl oz)
- Coconut oil (50ml; 2fl oz)
- Ghee (2 tbsp)
- Cider vinegar (20ml; ¾fl oz)
- Sherry vinegar (1 tbsp)
- Red wine vinegar (2 tbsp)
- Lime juice (1 tbsp)
- Lemon juice (225ml; 8fl oz)
- Coconut aminos (50ml; 2fl oz)
- Light coconut milk (1 litre; about 2 pints)
- Pumpkin purée (115g; 4oz)
- Maple syrup (50ml; 2fl oz)
- Unsweetened apple sauce (255g; 9oz)
- Honey (80ml; 3oz)
- Arrowroot powder (80g; 3oz)
- Coconut flour (2 tbsp)
- Bicarbonate of soda (2 tsp)
- Sea salt (1½ tsp)

Spices and Others

- Smoked sea salt (¼ tsp)
- Garlic powder (2¼ tsp)
- Onion powder (2 tsp)
- Dried oregano (1⅛ tsp)
- Dried thyme (⅛ tsp)
- Dried dill (½ tsp)
- Dried coriander (1 tsp)
- Dried basil (1 tsp)
- Turmeric (1½ tsp)
- Ground cloves (½ tsp)
- Cinnamon (2½ tsp)
- Ground ginger (1 tsp)
- Cream of tartar (1 tsp)
- Vanilla extract (1 tsp)
- Bacon fat (1 tbsp)
- White wine (50ml; 2fl oz)
- Pineapple juice (125ml; 4fl oz)
- Orange juice (50ml; 2fl oz)
- Unsweetened shredded coconut (30g; 1oz)
- Raisins (375g; 13oz)
- Dried cranberries (40g; 1½oz)
- Apricot preserves (60g; 2¼ oz)

Week 6 Meal Plan

	SUNDAY	MONDAY	TUESDAY
BREAKFAST	Sweet & Spicy Gra'no'la	Apple Cinnamon Hearts Cereal	Sweet & Spicy Gra'no'la
LUNCH	Spring Asparagus and Broccoli Soup	Spring Asparagus and Broccoli Soup	Mexican Carnitas Broth Bowl
DINNER	Mexican Carnitas Broth Bowl	Mexican Carnitas Broth Bowl	Lemon-Stuffed Sea Bass; Garlic Caper Roasted Cauliflower

Shopping List

Proteins
- Prawns, peeled and deveined (450g; 1lb)
- Whole sea bass, cleaned (about 1kg; 2kg)
- Salmon fillet, skin on (450g; 1lb)
- Duck breast, skin on (450g; 1lb))
- Boneless pork shoulder (1.6kg/3½lb)
- Pancetta (55g/2oz)

Produce
- Red onion (1)
- Shallot (1 large)
- Garlic (17 cloves)
- White onion (1)
- Green onions (4)
- Leeks (2 large)
- Parsley (15g; ½oz)
- Fresh coriander (35g; 1¼oz)
- Fresh thyme (4 tbsp + ½ tsp)

- Butternut squash (1 medium)
- Chayote or similar squash (1 medium)
- Rosemary (5 sprigs)
- Carrots (4–5)
- Rocket (50g; 2oz)
- Cauliflower (1 head)
- Asparagus (450g; 1lb)
- Broccoli (1 small head)

- Jicama or crisp apple (1 small)
- Avocados (2)
- Lemon (2)
- Limes (4)
- Mango (1)
- Orange (1)

WEDNESDAY	THURSDAY	FRIDAY	SATURDAY
Apple Cinnamon Hearts Cereal	Sweet & Spicy Gra'no'la	Apple Cinnamon Hearts Cereal	Sweet & Spicy Gra'no'la
Citrus Prawn Ceviche	Lemon-Stuffed Sea Bass; Garlic Caper Roasted Cauliflower	Citrus Prawn Ceviche	Spring Asparagus and Broccoli Soup
Roast Duck with Shallots, Figs, and Honey; Cinnamon Hasselback Sweet Potatoes	Maple Balsamic Glazed Salmon; Savoury Baked Butternut Squash	Roast Duck with Shallots, Figs, and Honey; Cinnamon Hasselback Sweet Potatoes	Maple Balsamic Glazed Salmon; Savoury Baked Butternut Squash

Store Cupboard

- Olive oil (175ml; 6fl oz)
- Coconut oil (80ml; 3fl oz)
- Coconut butter (1 tbsp)
- Cider vinegar (50ml; 2fl oz)
- Balsamic vinegar (50ml; 2fl oz)
- Lemon juice (80ml; 3fl oz)
- Lime juice (225ml; 8fl oz)
- Vegetable stock (600ml; 1 pint)
- Chicken stock (1 litre; 1½ pints)
- Capers (2 tbsp)
- Maple syrup (125ml; 4fl oz)
- Unsweetened apple sauce (250g; 9oz)
- Molasses (1 tbsp)
- Honey (2 tbsp)
- Light coconut milk (225ml; 8fl oz)
- Coconut flour (55g; 2oz)
- Arrowroot powder (65g; 2½oz)

Spices and Others

- Sea salt (2½ tsp)
- Dried oregano (1 tbsp + 1 tsp)
- Cinnamon (3 tsp)
- Onion powder (1½ tsp)
- Garlic powder (1½ tsp)
- Powdered turmeric (1½ tsp)
- Dried coriander (1 tsp)
- Dried basil (1 tsp)
- Dried dill (½ tsp)
- Ground ginger (½ tsp)
- Ground cloves (¼ tsp)
- Vanilla extract (2 tsp)
- Unsweetened coconut flakes (150g; 5½oz)
- Coconut sugar (½ tsp)
- Dried figs (150g; 5½oz)
- Unsweetened banana chips (55g; 2oz)
- Bacon fat (2 tbsp)
- Dry white wine (125ml; 4fl oz)
- Red wine (125ml; 4fl oz)

Glossary

arrowroot   A starch extracted from the roots of the arrowroot plant.

artichoke heart   The centre of the artichoke flower, often sold canned or frozen.

bake   To cook in a dry oven.

baking powder   A dry ingredient used to increase volume and lighten or leaven baked goods.

balsamic vinegar   A heavy, dark, sweet vinegar produced primarily in Italy from a specific type of grape and aged in wood barrels.

basil   A flavourful, almost sweet, resinous herb delicious with tomatoes and used in many Italian- and Mediterranean-style dishes.

baste   To keep foods moist during cooking by applying a liquid.

beat   To quickly mix substances.

blanch   To place a food in boiling water for about a minute to partially cook and then douse with cool water to halt the cooking.

blend   To completely mix something, usually with a blender or food processor; slower than beating.

boil   To heat a liquid to the point at which water turns into steam, causing the liquid to bubble. Also to cook food in boiling water.

bok choi   A member of the cabbage family with thick stems, crisp texture, and fresh flavour. Perfect for stir-frying.

braise   To cook with the introduction of a liquid, usually over a period of time.

broth   See stock.

brown   To cook in a frying pan, turning, until the food's surface is seared and brown in colour.

butternut squash   A bell-shaped winter squash with sweet orange-yellow flesh.

caper   The flavourful bud of a Mediterranean plant that is preserved in salt or vinegar.

caramelize   To cook vegetables or meat in butter or oil over a low heat until they soften, sweeten, and develop a caramel colour. Also to cook sugar over low heat until it develops a sweet caramel flavour.

ceviche   A seafood dish marinated for hours in lemon or lime juice, tomato, onion, and fresh coriander. The acidic citrus juice "cooks" the seafood.

chayote squash   A gourd with a pear-like shape, pale lime-green colour, sweet flavour, and crispy texture.

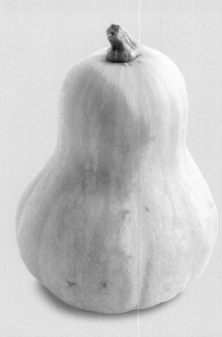

chiffonade   A chopping technique that involves shredding leafy vegetables into thin, ribbon-like pieces.

chive   A herb that grows in bunches of long leaves and offers a light onion flavour.

chop   To cut into pieces, usually qualified such as "coarsely chopped" or with a size measurement such as "chopped into 1.25cm (½-inch) pieces". "Finely chopped" is much closer to mince.

chutney   A thick condiment often served with Indian curries made with fruits and/or vegetables with vinegar, sugar, and spices.

cider vinegar   A vinegar produced from fermented apple juice.

carob   The flesh of tropical tree pods that are dried, baked, and powdered for use in baking. The flavour is similar to chocolate.

celeriac   A turnip-rooted celery variety with a knobby exterior and mild, crunchy flesh.

cinnamon   A rich, aromatic spice commonly used in baking or desserts.

clam juice   The liquid strained from freshly shucked clams. It has a briny fresh-fish taste that is used in many seafood dishes.

clove   A sweet, strong, almost wintergreen-flavoured spice used in baking.

coconut aminos   A soya-free seasoning (similar in flavour to soy sauce) made by fermenting coconut tree sap.

coconut butter   A thick and smooth butter made from the flesh of the coconut. It is thicker and richer than coconut oil.

coconut flour   A soft, dense flour derived from dried, ground coconut meat.

coconut milk   A milk made from one part shredded coconut and one part water. Coconut milk comes in full-fat and light varieties.

coconut oil   An oil extracted from the meat of the coconut fruit.

coconut sugar   A sugar produced from the liquid sap of cut flower buds of the coconut palm tree.

coriander   A member of the parsley family often used in Mexican dishes. The seed is called coriander; in North America, the plant is called cilantro.

count   In terms of seafood or other foods that come in small sizes, the number of the item that compose 450g (1 lb).

cremini mushroom   A brown, richly flavoured mushroom. The larger, fully grown version is the portobello.

curry powder   A blend of rich and flavourful spices such as hot pepper, nutmeg, cumin, cinnamon, pepper, and turmeric.

dash   A few drops, usually of a liquid, released by a quick shake.

dates   A sweet dried fruit with a large inedible pit.

deglaze   To scrape up bits of meat and seasonings left in a pan after cooking, usually by adding a liquid such as wine or stock, to create a flavourful stock.

dehydrator   An appliance that circulates warm air around food to encourage the evaporation of its water content.

devein   To remove the dark vein from the back of a large shrimp with a sharp knife.

dice   To cut into small cubes about 5mm (¼ inch) square.

dill   A herb perfect for eggs, salmon, cheese dishes, and vegetables.

dredge   To coat a piece of food on all sides with a dry substance such as flour or cornmeal.

emulsion   A combination of liquid ingredients carefully and quickly beaten together to create a thick liquid, such as a fat or oil with water.

endive   A green that resembles a small, elongated, tightly packed head of romaine lettuce. The thick, crunchy leaves can be broken off and used with dips and spreads.

extra-virgin olive oil   See olive oil.

extract   A concentrated flavouring derived from foods or plants through evaporation or distillation that imparts a powerful flavour without altering the volume or texture of a dish.

fennel   In seed form, a fragrant, liquorice-tasting herb. The bulbs have a mild flavour and a celery-like crunch.

figs   A small, soft, pear-shaped fruit with a sweet, seedy flesh that can be eaten fresh or dried.

fish sauce   A Thai and Vietnamese sauce known for its savory, sweet, and umami flavours that is extracted from fermented anchovies.

fold   To combine a dense and a light mixture with a gentle move from the middle of the bowl outward to preserve the mixture's airy nature.

fry   See sauté.

frying pan   A flat-bottomed metal pan with a handle designed to cook food on a hob.

garlic   A pungent and flavourful member of the onion family. A garlic bulb contains multiple cloves; each clove, when chopped, yields about 1 teaspoon garlic.

gelatine   A substance derived from the collagen of animal by-products (skin, tendons, ligaments, and bones) that is commonly used in the production of jellies.

ghee   A clarified butter made by heating butter to separate and remove the milk solids.

ginger   A flavourful root available fresh or dried and ground that adds a pungent, sweet, and spicy quality to a dish.

golden raisin   A raisin made from a white grape.

grill   To cook under the overhead high-heat element.

hearts of palm   Firm, elongated, off-white cylinders from the inside of a palm tree stem tip.

horseradish   A sharp, spicy root that can be grated and prepared as a condiment.

infusion   A liquid in which flavourful ingredients such as herbs have been steeped to extract their flavour into the liquid.

Italian seasoning   A blend of dried herbs, including basil, oregano, rosemary, and thyme.

jicama   A large, round vegetable that's juicy, crunchy, and sweet. If you can't find jicama, substitute sliced water chestnuts or a tart green apple.

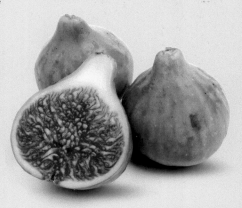

julienne A French word meaning "to slice into very thin pieces".

kalamata olive Traditionally from Greece, a medium-small, long, black olive with a rich, smoky flavour.

Key lime A very small lime grown primarily in Florida known for its tart taste.

kosher salt A coarse-grained salt made without additives or iodine.

leeks A long cylindrical vegetable resembling an oversized spring onion with a sweet onion flavour.

marinate To soak a food in a seasoned sauce to impart flavour and make tender, as with meat.

marjoram A sweet herb similar to oregano, popular in Greek, Spanish, and Italian dishes.

mesclun Mixed salad greens such as lettuce, arugula, cress, and endive.

mince To cut into very small pieces, smaller than diced, about 3mm (1/8 inch) or smaller.

monkfish A bottom-dwelling anglerfish with a meaty texture and mild taste.

olive The green or black fruit of the olive tree.

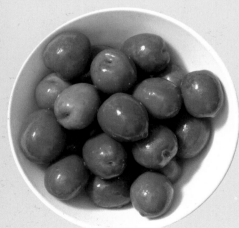

olive oil A fragrant liquid produced by crushing or pressing olives. Extra-virgin olive oil, the most flavourful and highest quality, is produced from the olives' first pressing; oil is also produced from later pressings.

oregano A fragrant, slightly astringent herb used often in Greek, Spanish, and Italian dishes.

oxidation The gradual browning of a fruit or vegetable from exposure to air. Minimize oxidation by rubbing cut surfaces with lemon juice.

pancetta A salt-cured Italian bacon made from pork belly.

parboil To partially cook in boiling water or broth.

parsley A fresh-tasting green leafy herb, often used as a garnish.

parsnip A root vegetable that closely resembles a carrot, but with a white colour and mild sweet flavour.

pâté A mixture of cooked ground meat and fat minced together into a spreadable paste.

pesto A thick spread or sauce made with pine nuts, fresh basil, garlic, olive oil, and Parmesan cheese.

portobello mushroom A large, brown, chewy, flavourful mushroom.

preheat To turn on an oven, grill, or other cooking appliance early so it will be hot when the dish is ready to be cooked.

prosciutto A dry-cured ham that is typically very thinly sliced.

purée To reduce a food to a thick, creamy texture, typically using a blender or food processor.

purple sweet potato A variety of sweet potato with a deep-purple skin and vibrant purple flesh.

pinch An unscientific measurement for the amount of an ingredient you can hold between your finger and thumb.

poach To cook a food in simmering liquid such as water, wine, or broth.

reduce To boil or simmer a broth or sauce to remove some of the water content and yield a more concentrated flavour.

reserve To hold a specified ingredient for use later in a recipe.

rocket A spicy, peppery green that has a sharp, distinctive flavour.

roast To cook food uncovered in an oven, usually without additional liquid.

rosemary A pungent, sweet herb used with chicken, pork, fish, and especially lamb.

sage An herb with a slightly musty, fruity, lemon-rind scent and earthy flavour.

sauté To pan-cook over lower heat than what's used for frying.

scallops Marine bivalve molluscs. Scallops come in a variety of sizes, including large sea scallops and small bay scallops.

sear To quickly brown the exterior of a food, especially meat, over high heat.

shallot A member of the onion family that grows in a bulb. Similar to garlic, but with a milder onion flavour.

shellfish A broad range of seafood, including clams, mussels, oysters, crabs, shrimp, and lobster.

shiitake mushroom A large, dark-brown mushroom with a hearty, meaty flavour.

simmer To boil gently so the liquid barely bubbles.

skim To remove fat or other material from the top of liquid.

smoked sea salt A sea salt that has been naturally smoked over wood fires and gives a smoky aroma and flavour to food.

spaghetti squash A winter squash with a bright yellow shell and a sweet flesh that, when cooked, resembles the texture and appearance of spaghetti noodles.

spiralize A method of cutting vegetables using a spiralizer which carves long, thin, noodle-like pieces from vegetables.

steam To suspend a food over boiling water and allow the heat of the steam to cook the food.

steep To set something a liquid, as in steeping tea in hot water.

stew To slowly cook pieces of food submerged in a liquid. Also a dish prepared using this method.

stir-fry To cook small pieces of food in a wok or skillet over high heat, moving and turning the food quickly to cook all sides.

stock A flavourful broth made by cooking meats and/or vegetables with seasonings until the liquid absorbs these flavours. The stock is strained, and the solids are discarded. Stock can be eaten alone or used as a base for soups, stews, etc.

swede A root vegetable with yellow flesh and a flavour similar to a turnip.

tapioca A starchy white flour extracted from the cassava plant.

tarragon A sweet, rich-smelling herb perfect with vegetables, seafood, chicken, and pork.

tartar sauce A mayonnaise-based sauce often used as a condiment with seafood dishes.

Tenderstem broccoli A hybrid of broccoli and kale with slender stalks and small florets.

thyme A minty, zesty herb.

turmeric A spicy, pungent yellow root. It's the source of the yellow colour in many mustards.

vegetable steamer A perforated insert designed to fit in or on a saucepan to hold food to be s teamed above boiling water.

vinaigrette A light salad dressing made with oil, vinegar, and seasonings.

vinegar An acidic liquid often made from fermented grapes, apples, or rice and used as a dressing and seasoning.

wasabi A Japanese plant that tastes like strong horseradish and is used in a powder or paste form.

water chestnut A white, crunchy, juicy tuber popular in many Asian dishes.

whisk To mix rapidly, introducing air to the mixture.

white mushroom A button mushroom with an earthy smell and appealing soft crunch.

white vinegar Vinegar produced from grain.

wine vinegar Vinegar produced from red or white wine.

zest Small slivers of peel, usually from citrus fruit.

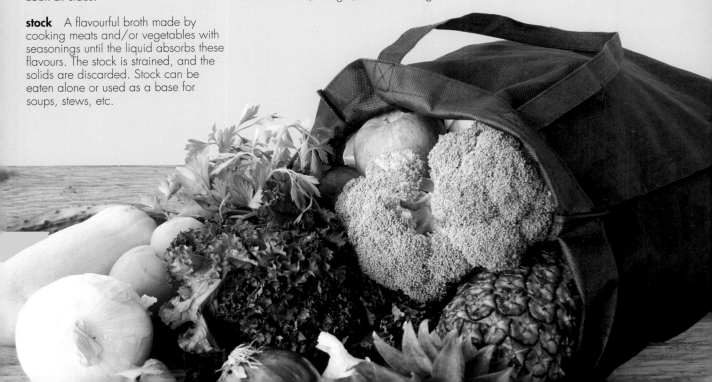

Index

All photography by Amari Thomsen, with the following exceptions:

p14 Andy Crawford © Dorling Kindersley
p14 Chris Villano © Dorling Kindersley
p14 David Murray © Dorling Kindersley
p15 David Murray and Jules Selmes
     © Dorling Kindersley
p19 Lorenzo Vecchia © Dorling Kindersley

p29 Sian Irvine © Dorling Kindersley
p29 Gaby Cheikh © Dorling Kindersley
p52 Dave King © Dorling Kindersley
p177 William Reavell © Dorling Kindersley
p214 Dave King © Dorling Kindersley
p215 Philip Dowell © Dorling Kindersley

p216 Lorenzo Vecchia © Dorling Kindersley
p217 Stuart West © Dorling Kindersley
p217 Will Heap © Dorling Kindersley
p218 Lorenzo Vecchia © Dorling Kindersley